The Energy Break

Also by Bradford Keeney, Ph.D.

Everyday Soul: Awakening the Spirit in Daily Life

Improvisational Therapy: A Practical Guide for Creative Clinical Strategies

The Therapeutic Voice of Olga Silverstein

Mind in Therapy

Aesthetics of Change

The Energy Break
Recharge Your Life with Autokinetics

Bradford Keeney, Ph.D.

Golden Books

New York

Golden Books®
888 Seventh Avenue
New York, NY 10106

Designed by Marc Burckhardt
Illustrations by András Halasz
Manufactured in the United States of America

10 9 8 7 6 5 4 3 2 1

Library of Congress Cataloging-in-Publication Data

Keeney, Bradford P.
   The energy break : recharge your life with autokinetics /
Bradford Keeney.
      p.   cm.
   Includes bibliographical references.
   ISBN 0-307-44036-2 (alk. paper)
   1. Relaxation.   2. Stress management.   3. Vitality.   4. Fatigue-Prevention.
I. Title.   II. Title: Simple technique to help you with everyday fatigue, low energy
& lack of vitality.
RA785.K44   1998
613.7—dc21
                                                              97-26900
                                                                  CIP

To Marian and Scott

ACKNOWLEDGMENTS

I am grateful to all the indigenous teachers and traditional healers throughout the world who taught me about bringing the universal life force into our daily lives. They have encouraged me to share this knowledge with you, and I do so with great enthusiasm and respect for the traditions that have preserved these energy practices for thousands of years. In particular, I am deeply appreciative to the Kalahari Bushmen, who brought me into their family; to the Guarani elders, who ordained this work; to Vusumazulu Credo Mutwa, the Zulu High Sanusi, for his initiation and teaching; and to the great Japanese healer, Ikuko Osumi, Sensei, for her steadfast support and inspiration.

I am especially thankful for the prodigious way in which Laura Yorke, Bob Asahina, Cassie Jones, and Lara Asher at Golden Books guided the making of this book. I also want to thank my incredibly talented literary agent, Arielle Eckstut; the folks at James Levine Communications; and my lecture agent, Kitty Farmer, and her colleague, Dana Roberts, for their many wonderful contributions to helping me get the word out. And a special acknowledgment to Nancy Connor and the Ringing Rocks Foundation for the many ways in which they help preserve idigenous healing traditions.

Finally, deepest love and appreciation to my wife, Marian, and my son, Scott, for their patience and enthusiasm at every step of this work.

CONTENTS

Introduction
Discovering the Secret of an Energized Life   1

Chapter One
Why We Get Tired   13

Chapter Two
The Three-Step Technique   39

Chapter Three
Entering the Charged Life   73

Protecting Yourself from the Energy Drain
Activating the Inborn Ability to Heal Yourself
Experiencing Healing
A Moving Meditation
How Life Energy Changes Your Diet
Beyond Exercise as You Now Know It
Finding Effective Ways to Solve Your Problems
Awakening Your Personal Creativity
Skinship with Others:
The Art of Revitalizing Your Intimate Relationships by Touching
Discovering the Ancient Mysteries of Life
Energized Prayer

Chapter Four
The Twelve Questions Most Often Asked   135

Chapter Five
Life Energy in Ancient and Modern Traditions   141

Suggested Reading   181

About the Author   187

INTRODUCTION

Discovering the Secret of an Energized Life

Do you continually fight the battle of fatigue? Are you tired of not having the vitality you want in the most important moments of your life? Does your life sometimes feel as if it is slipping away because you don't have the energy to be fully engaged in it?

Whether you are trying to get out of bed in the morning, fighting to stay awake during an important meeting, mobilizing your concentration to get a job done, or pushing yourself to be alert as you drive home from work, the fight against low energy shows up in every aspect of our daily lives.

Although we have become a health-conscious generation that values the importance of diet, exercise, and relaxation, we still struggle to have more vitality and energy. We have learned how to trim our thighs and abdomen, increase the distance we can jog, and lower the level of our cholesterol, but we are still plagued by flare-ups of fatigue that can strike at any time. Perhaps you have a stand-up job—like a waitress, factory worker, doctor, or salesclerk—and you want to learn a way to stay on your feet, and stay vibrant, through the course of your daily work. Or you may have a desk job and know all too well that sitting is also tiring work. Standing or sitting, moving or staying still, we get worn out and come face to face with one of the biggest problems of our time: how to get the energy and vitality to make it through each day.

It's not only the workplace that brings these challenges to energy. When we go home to our families or meet with our friends, we often find that we could use a boost of energy to optimize our time with them. Our spouses, our friends, and particularly our children can wear us out, and when we become exhausted we are susceptible to feeling low and depressed. Although we want to give our best to them, most of us feel that we need some kind of break that can energize and vitalize us to be at our peak performance with those we care the most about.

We desperately need more than a coffee break or a moment of relaxation. All of us—women and men, young and old—are looking for a way to easily and quickly recharge ourselves: a true energy break.

Such a practice already exists. It is a simple technique that is available to you, and you are about to discover it. By following a simple set of instructions, you will be able to experience and nurture energy in your daily life. You can finally shed your everyday fatigue, low energy, and lack of vitality *in a matter of minutes.*

It is my great fortune to bring you this gift, and I promise it will change your life forever. As someone who has taught psychotherapy for nearly twenty years, I am well aware that some people are reluctant to try anything new. With respect to this work, I can assure you that I have met all kinds of people, including some who came to me with great trepidation about learning this skill. But to their great surprise and delight, they found that it literally took no effort to learn how to energize their lives.

I will be up front with you: What I have to teach you requires no complicated understanding or special indoctrination. It is a simple, natural, effortless practice that you can begin immediately. As you will discover, you have held this knowledge inside you from the moment you were born, but it has been hidden. My job is to lead you back to this natural resource, one of the most remarkable gifts ever given to you, so that you may use it to energize and enhance your everyday life.

The Ocean of Life Energy

To receive this gift you must first understand that we live in a universal ocean of life energy. Although we can't see this ocean, it is every bit as real as the one that dolphins, whales, and fish inhabit. Like the sea, our ocean surrounds us with many streams, eddies, and currents. But instead of water, the currents in our ocean consist of energy. This energy is the *universal life force.*

Whether you are at the workplace, in your home, or on the tennis court, you are always in this ocean of energy. You were born to take in its energy regularly in order to stay full of vitality. Unfortunately, most of us have forgotten how to do this. Our situation is analogous to trying to get through each day with only one breath. Imagine getting up in the morning, taking in one big breath, and then trying to hold it throughout the day, hoping you will have enough air to sustain you until you go to sleep again. As impossible as this may sound, it is what most people try to do with life energy. During their evening sleep they take a breath of energy to get them through the next day, and then they find themselves gasping for more vitality as they move through their daily activities. It is time for you to stop trying to live each day with a single breath of energy. Just as it takes no work to breathe in the air you need, it takes no effort to bring in the energy required to live an optimal life. Introduce yourself to the simple practice of drawing this life force into you.

When we are vibrantly alive, the currents of energy from the ocean of life flow through us in an effortless, natural way. When the currents flow smoothly in and out of us we become a revitalizing fountain of life energy, like a *fountain of youth*—the dynamic source of youthful vitality sought by explorers throughout the ages. This life-nourishing fountain does not exist only in some exotic foreign land. It is found in the unique movements of your body that bring the life force through you.

Global Recognition of Life Energy

For centuries, people from China to Africa have called upon special movements of the body that bring in the energy of life. Every ancient tradition around the world has its own name for this life energy. It is called *chi* or *qi* in China, *ki* in Japan, *num* among the Kalahari Bushmen, *tumpinyeri mooroop* in Aboriginal Australia, *prana* in India, *yesod* by Jewish cabalists, *holy spirit* by Christians, *baraka* by Sufis, *manitou* by the Ojibway, and *ha* in Hawaii. Among many indigenous people it is often simply referred to as *medicine.*

As a university professor who has written extensively on psychotherapy, I had the opportunity to travel around the world giving speeches and teaching classes. During my travels I took the time to visit some of the oldest healing cultures on earth—including the Kalahari Bushmen of Africa and the Aborigines of Australia—and diverse indigenous elders throughout North and South America. I worked with traditional healers, shamans, medicine people, and revered teachers who shared the heart and essence of their ancient wisdom. In my travels I lived with one of the greatest healers of our time, Ikuko Osumi, Sensei, a revered elder woman in Tokyo. Her clients include many of the leaders of old and new Japan, from master teachers of the ancient Japanese arts to executives of Japan's leading industries. From Osumi, Sensei, I learned what all these teachers from around the world commonly hold as their most powerful practice: it is the practice of bringing the universal life force into our physical bodies to energize and revitalize our lives on a daily basis.

The practical technique I will present to you is directly based upon their secret of working with the life force.

My involvement with these global healing traditions changed my life. I learned firsthand how to have a direct experience of life energy—a direct contact. And after seeing the quick and often dramatic changes in clients that are brought about by this energy work, I devoted myself to working with the life force. I was no longer able to practice conventional forms of psychotherapy. I retired from the university, left my academic practice of family therapy, and began teaching others how to draw upon the natural energy of life.

Energy Can Transform Your Life

When you enter more deeply into the ocean of life energy, you will be amazed to find how every aspect of your daily life is revitalized and transformed. You may find, among other outcomes, these new possibilities:

- Finding ways to successfully avoid the energy drain.
- Developing your inborn ability to heal yourself and thereby opening the door to the world of natural healing and its inexhaustable offerings.
- Uncovering why meditation doesn't work for some people, and the secret to making it work for you.

- Discovering a new way to orient yourself toward dieting—having a flexible diet that changes with the natural flow of your life.
- Creating a true alternative to daily workouts, an alternative in which you discover physical exercise that is painless and natural.
- Tapping into an oasis of solutions to the difficulties and challenges of everyday life.
- Bringing forth the flow of more creativity in your daily activities.
- Revitalizing and recharging your personal and intimate relationships, including a powerful new form of sexuality.
- Awakening direct access to and connection with the deepest mysteries of life.

The benefits of circulating the life force through your whole being are greater than those you would find if you tried every health spa, therapy, medicine, and health practice in the world. Indeed, the oldest and most powerful medicine, as Hippocrates acknowledged, is found in the force of life itself. It alone has the power to energize, vitalize, and even heal your life. All practices and techniques that provide you with any help do so because they indirectly bring some life force to you. The alternative presented here is for you to go straight to the source.

Getting That Extra Boost of Energy: A Story About a Young Gymnast

Here's a story about a young woman I met last year. What happened to her demonstrates the power of the life force to overcome the impasses and difficulties that sometimes block your forward progress.

I received a call from this woman's mother, a researcher at the

Mayo Clinic in Rochester, Minnesota. She said that her daughter was a competitive college gymnast who had received knee surgery several years ago. Although the best doctors at the Mayo Clinic had worked with her, they were startled to find that after she recovered from surgery she was unable to perform a forward somersault. She was sent to various departments throughout the clinic, from surgery to physical rehabilitation to psychiatry. Among other things, her therapists made her a personalized audiocassette that guided her through some visualization exercises before her gymnastic routine.

No matter what they tried, nothing worked. For several years, she found herself unable to move every time she attempted a forward somersault. The Mayo Clinic gave up and suggested that perhaps she should try some alternative approach, such as hypnosis. The girl's parents subsequently went on a search to find an alternative treatment for their daughter and were given the name of the Milton Erickson Foundation in Phoenix, Arizona, a center world-renowned for hypnosis and innovative work in psychotherapy. After the director of the foundation listened to their story, he recommended that they have a meeting with me.

When the young gymnast, now a college student in Wisconsin, came to my house, I told her about the universal life force and demonstrated the three-step technique that I describe in Chapter Two. I then brought the life force into her knee and suggested that she start moving her body in a way that would draw the life force into her whole being. After one week of doing this, she returned to me and said that she had felt a tingling in her knee throughout the week, and that to her great surprise, and her coach's surprise, she had spontaneously done a double somersault during a practice session. One week of recharging herself was able to bring forth what years of medical treatment were unable to accomplish. She is now a regular practitioner of this simple technique and has found the fountain that energizes her, bringing vitality to her gymnastics and her daily life.

No miracle took place in the gymnast's recovery of her ability to spring forward into a somersault. All she did was move with the currents of life's ocean of energy. When this occurred, her life and body moved forward in a natural, spontaneous way. This revitalization of energy is available to you at any time.

Do you dream of being able to effortlessly scale new heights in your day-to-day life? Everyone knows what it is like to run toward a goal, but to be stopped in your tracks because you were missing that extra something that could lift you to the top. What you need to ascend to the height of life is a boost from life itself, the force that is capable of moving you toward realizing your dreams and aspirations.

Give Yourself an Energy Break

But the life energy that is freely available to you can do more than help you achieve your biggest goals. It is also present to help you through all of the nitty-gritty details of daily life. Whether it's washing the dishes, changing the baby's diapers, filling out your income tax forms, or getting enough energy to be your best for a business meeting, a family trip, or an evening date, life awaits your tapping into its endless reservoir of revitalizing energy. It is time that you do more than take a coffee (or tea) break. Start giving yourself an *energy break,* and discover the joy of transcending the barrier of tiredness. Find out how easy and natural it is to bring the energy in and live each day with fresh vitality.

I have taught businessmen how to get energized before giving a sales pitch. When filled with energy, they exude natural charisma and find that their ideas are more readily received and accepted. The key to having this competitive edge is simply taking an energy break minutes before starting a business presentation. I have also worked with mothers who took an energy break to help their babies go back to sleep in the middle of the night. By rocking the baby in a special way, the mother becomes revitalized while the baby calms down. Every age group can benefit from this practice, from crawling infants to career-climbing adults to those in the midst of their golden years. I have found that energy breaks are especially useful to retired people, who can draw upon them to recharge their daily lives and bring forth creative ideas and enthusiasm for everyday life.

What is this energy break that promises to transform your life? It involves an amazingly simple technique called *Autokinetics*, referring to the practice of making automatic, effortless body movements that bring forth the life force. Your body is already wired to do these movements, and they will take place automatically when you learn how to trigger them. It is simply a matter of turning on the switch that releases this innate body response. Anyone can learn to do Autokinetics. It is as easy as sitting in a rocking chair and allowing yourself to gently rock back and forth.

With Autokinetics, you bring a true energy break into your life. As children, we were given a recess during the school day, a time when we could be free from the purposeful effort of schoolwork. As adults we lost our recess, and this loss has taken its toll on our health and well being. In the most general sense, Autokinetics is the practice of effortless action, and in this regard it is a pure recess. It teaches you how to do less in order to have more. It frees you from having to follow the perfect diet, exercise program, meditation teacher, lifestyle consultant, weekly psychotherapist, or spiritual guide. Instead, you learn how to bring forth energizing resonances with the food you eat, the physical motions you make, the thoughts and feelings you have, and the ways you move toward living each day.

The Energy Way of Life

The energy orientation changes everything. First of all, you will be able to retire from all the hard work that it takes to make yourself healthy and happy. The cost of this hard work is that it makes your life too unnatural, forceful, and purposeful, taking you away from the most satisfying way you can live. In other words, you drift away from effortless living, the truest sign of a vibrant life.

As you will learn, the secret to optimizing your state of well-being is rolling with the punches of life. When people who have lived past 100 years of age are interviewed, researchers find that their diet, exercise, and lifestyle aren't necessarily associated with their longevity. There are plenty of strong, healthy aged people who curse, smoke, drink whiskey, and get wild. Their testimony goes against the grain of what most health experts say is good for you. The only factor that ever stands out clearly and consistently is the fact that these people don't let life get them out of whack. They don't overworry about the bad things that happen to them but are able to roll with the punches that come their way. They provide a great example of what is most essential about maintaining health and longevity—they do not fight and resist life, but *move with it.* The message for you is to allow yourself to move with the energy that life brings. Literally move and dance your body through each day so that there are more days to your life, with each one being all that it possibly can be.

I've seen Autokinetics have profound effects—extending beyond simple vitality—on hundreds of people. I treated a middle-aged high school science teacher from Connecticut who suffered from asthmatic coughing, lack of energy, and the problems that come from being overweight. Although he was skeptical at first, after a week of taking ten-minute energy breaks with Autokinetics, he found that he could achieve an inner state of peace and relaxation that helped him reduce his asthmatic episodes. Furthermore, new inspiration came to him for his daily teaching, which in turn brought forth a new surge of energy and motivation. And finally, these positive experiences resulted in his being drawn to eat in a way that didn't lead to perpetuating his over-weight condition. He didn't go on any diet, but he found that the new tuning of his life brought forth a natural change in what he desired to eat. All these changes brought into his life new health and a powerful sense of feeling well.

A twenty-five-year-old woman in Miami who was beginning a ca-reer in advertising used Autokinetics and found that it gave her more than a daily energy boost. It also triggered moments of inspiration for designing advertising campaigns. When she took an energy break, she would sometimes get an idea that would inspire her work. She learned to use the flow of life energy for both her well-being and her career success.

A retired couple in Phoenix learned Autokinetics together, and they now use it to bring fresh vitality to their golden years. They start each morning with an energy break and find that it brings about a strong desire to meet the unique challenges and opportunities of the day. They call it their "time for dancing together" when they sit down in two chairs and do some natural movements together. Their friends and family, who at first thought that such a simple technique couldn't possibly bring about any noticeable change, now remark on the cou-ple's newfound healthy glow and enthusiastic spirit.

The *energy way of life* invites you to draw freely upon the energy and vitality that is present in every breath that you take. Rather than sitting around brooding over self-analysis and inner criticism, get off the therapist's couch and enter the playground of life energy. How can you expect to take the next step that you need to take if you are lying down or sitting still, drowning in your own whirling thoughts and emotions? Move yourself in order to move your life forward. Take a few moments to add an energy break to your daily life—a recess for initiating the simple practice of Autokinetics. Here you can naturally move yourself right into the life you have always desired and hoped was possible to achieve.

What I bring to you does not promise new understanding, insights, hypotheses, or theories that will change in the next year or even the next 100 years. What I bring you is, in my opinion, *the most vital wisdom of life itself*—the direct path to bringing new energy into your body, mind, and soul. This heartbeat of life—the rhythmical pulse of the universal life force—can be held in every pore of your being. Prepare to take a true energy break and embrace the movement that can energize, motivate, and recharge every aspect of your life.

CHAPTER ONE

Why We Get Tired

Today, in an age of downsizing, extended work hours, and chronic fatigue syndrome, our overriding concern is that we are too tired or simply do not have enough energy to get through the day effectively. Once we finally arrive at the office—after the kids are dropped off at school, the dry cleaning is brought in, and paychecks are deposited at the bank—we tank up on caffeine in order to make it to lunch. When it's time for lunch, we stuff food and caffeinated sodas into our system, hoping that by refueling our engine, we'll make it to the end of the day. But midafternoon arrives and the caffeine hasn't kicked in, so we reach for the sugar stash hidden in our desk drawers. No matter what we try, we feel drained of energy and become susceptible to falling into the quicksand of fatigue. As a result, our productivity and morale go down, and we take less and less enjoyment from both our work and our family life.

Have you ever been so fed up and discouraged by being worn out and fatigued that you went straight to a health food store and loaded up on vitamins, energy supplements, and herbal tonics that promised to rejuvenate you? Perhaps you dove into the latest fad diet, eating all the right vegetables and fruit juices. Perhaps you gave yourself extra hours of sleep in a crash attempt to revitalize yourself. Or maybe you purchased a newly designed pillow or relaxation tape that promised you a deeper slumber, and then signed up for the latest weekend course on meditation. What is perplexing about these attempted solutions is that even though they seem to be the right things to do, they usually don't get rid of your fatigue. What so many of us have discovered is that getting enough rest, maintaining a healthy diet, following an exercise program, meditating, and supplementing our daily regimen with numerous offerings from the health-conscious marketplace too often leave us feeling as tired as we were before.

The problem is that we have been taught that our body operates like a machine—when we run out of energy, we assume that we are low on fuel and need to fill ourselves up with something, whether it be food, vitamin supplements, or even a sugar treat. Unfortunately, when we refuel our internal tank, give our body engine a rest, or jog around the block, it is usually not enough to revitalize us and bring us back to an optimal energy state.

If our bodies were simply machines, then having the right intake would result in the optimal output. Eating the right diet, getting enough rest, and keeping the body in good shape would be the simple answer to having a vital life. But this doesn't always work. Clearly, the analogy of our bodies as machines is challenged by the facts of our everyday experience. Something is missing from our understanding of how we are supposed to manage our lives.

You must step beyond the limitations of this analogy—the body as a machine—and begin seeing yourself as a sensitive musical instrument: you experience well-being and harmony as long as you are kept *in tune.* In this chapter I will show that when the movements and rhythms of your body processes are in tune with the natural energies that surround you, you are open to receive this energy. However, when your body instrument goes out of tune, you feel drained of energy and become susceptible to what feels like inescapable fatigue.

Signs of Being Out of Tune

All of us, at one time or another, have the following experiences. You should pay more attention to them when they begin to take place and regard them as signs that you are in the midst of a process that is carrying you out of tune. When you are out of tune, it is natural to really feel out of whack. This can be experienced as anything from a mild sensation of imbalance to a strong sense of panic. Do not unnecessarily regard such experiences as deep-seated psychological problems that require professional help. Instead, consider whether you are presently out of tune with your life activities and surroundings. Do not overlook any of these discomforting experiences. They are strong indications that you need to find a way to bring yourself back into a naturally tuned state. Here are the signs that you are becoming out of tune:

• You spend too much time worrying, either about problems of the past or about anticipated difficulties of the future. Sometimes you feel this worry as a pain in your gut, a stiffness in your lower back or neck, or a tightness in your chest. You spend far too much energy being a psychotherapist, accountant, judge, advocate, and critic for the events of your life and the lives of those who are close to you.

• You dread an upcoming task, meeting, or activity. Again, you may feel this discomfort in your body. You may find yourself awakening in the middle of the night with a sense of deep dread that ruins the quality of your rest.

• You physically bump into things throughout the day, for no apparent reason. Whether it's the bedroom dresser, the refrigerator door, the hall wall, or the car door, your body seems off-balance and unsure of its place. You curse under your breath, since these little bumps bring unsettling bruises into your daily routines.

- You find it difficult to focus on what you are doing. Your mind wanders all over the place, usually stopping only momentarily, in your worries or else in some never-ending strategy for "making it all work out." You do everything in an incomplete way, never throwing your whole self into the task at hand.

- Almost everyone and everything easily irritates you. You know that you are too easily irritated by matters that shouldn't get to you, but you can't help it. It's as if someone wired you to respond robotically with irritation. You see it coming, can't stop it, and then there you are, an irritable mess. And that irritates you even more.

- You count the number of hours or days or weeks that must pass in order to get to the end of something that troubles you. Like the inmates in prison who mark off each day on the wall calendar, you seem to be waiting to escape the prison life has made especially for you. Unfortunately, no end seems in sight, and you don't even know where to go to get a pardon or an early release from doing your time.

- There's little excitement or anticipation of excitement in your everyday life. The biggest thrill is falling asleep on the couch after a hard day's work. You no longer look forward to going out or doing anything. You find yourself crawling from one couch or easy chair to another.

- You seldom think of pursuing any kind of happiness. It's absolutely impossible for you to imagine anything that could help your situation, short of winning the lottery. If you think that money is your only solution, then you're out of tune.

- You are tempted to believe that you never can quite win the victory you want, and you assume that you will always fall short of the mark. You don't feel like a winner; you feel like a second-class performer, a B-movie extra, or an unnoticed nerd. No matter what you try, you predict that you will lose.

• You are truly tired of being tired. Over time your tiredness becomes a superfatigue that seems to sink you deeper into exhaustion and an almost complete lack of vitality.

• Life in general feels unnatural, and it takes a lot of serious effort to move yourself through the day. You wonder if there is something wrong with your body because it simply takes too much work to get through your daily activities, much less your week. You're wondering whether you have chronic fatigue syndrome.

• You're beginning to think about seeing a psychiatrist to get medication that will make you feel better. How could the side effects be any worse than what you feel already?

• You can't imagine anyone else seeing you as filled with energy and vitality. You fear that you sometimes look like death warmed over.

• Life seems like a painful obstacle course. Everywhere you look, there is something that tries to trip you or knock you down. There are no downhill glides, only uphill challenges. Why can't you find a slope to coast on? Why is everything a major mountain to cross?

• You have stopped fantasizing. You've become so worn down from everyday life that you've given up your dreams. You no longer tell anyone about your latest ideas, projects, hopes, or inspirations. You simply complain all the time and go on and on about how awful your life has become. You feel as though any luck that might have once been available has passed you by. You may even wonder if you are cursed.

• You are becoming cynical about anyone else's happiness, joy, enthusiasm, or vitality. You're convinced that other people's happiness is not real, but only an illusion that makes their lives a complete lie. If you can't feel any energy in your life, then why not deny that it even exists? You know that science will prove that nothing works anyway.

• You care less about the world than you did as a young person. Idealism was wasted on your youth. You can't imagine the zeal you once had for changing the world. You can't find a way to vitalize your own life, let alone send some energy into the bigger systems that have been stuck for decades or centuries.

• You enjoy watching news reports about disasters more than you enjoy hearing an old-fashioned story that celebrates the joy of living. Nothing like seeing someone else having a worse situation than your own. Gives you a moment of relief. But it's too much to see that Pollyanna stuff that makes you feel worse about your own uninspiring situation.

• Everything about your general state of being feels off-course. You don't have a clue as to what direction your compass is pointing in. It's probably even worse: you've lost your compass and the ability to distinguish one direction from another. You scare yourself by the reckless ways in which you are tempted to roam.

• You talk about spirituality, but your life lacks spirit. Whether you thump the Bible or shout the truth of New Age testimony, you talk the talk but don't walk the walk. It's become more a matter of showing that you really have the truth.

• There is little mystery in your life. The only mystery left is why anyone could possibly be mystified by anything. The magic has slipped away, and you wish you could feel enough energy to try anything new just one more time.

If you have had any one of these experiences, it is likely that you have been seriously out of tune at one point or another, or chronically. Instead of taking another step in the same direction, prepare to orient yourself for a tuning. Even if you are experiencing many of these symptoms, give yourself a chance to become tuned, energized, and revitalized before you become overly dependent upon psychotherapeutic intervention.

Signs of Being in Tune

On the other hand, recall those times when you were passionately engrossed in a major project. It may have been planting an inspired garden plot, redecorating your house, performing a special task at work, or helping your child with a school paper. No matter what the focus of the project, if you completely throw yourself into it with untempered enthusiasm and absolute dedication, you feel totally energized. Remarkably enough, you receive this energy and vitality even if you don't pay attention to any of those things we are told are necessary for our well-being.

All of us have had times when we were well tuned and charged by the natural flow of the universal life force. Following are descriptions of what it is like to be tuned, in this completely natural way. Whenever you perceive yourself having any of these experiences, do not stay too long in the position of observing yourself. This will remove you from the flow of the experience and tempt you to spend too much time speculating on it, or accounting for it through some form of psychological or spiritual explanation, or simply gloating too much over your own success, all of which could bring you out of tune again. Simply accept these experiences as a natural consequence of being tuned.

• Your body movements feel natural. Whether you are walking along a sidewalk, getting ready to sit down, or bending over to pick up a pencil, these everyday movements take place with a sense of natural grace and rhythm. A walk across the street can give you the same satisfaction that a successfully executed three-point shot or slam dunk gives to an NBA basketball player.

- You seldom worry, but often feel joy, excitement, and enthusiastic anticipation about your life. For example, you know this experience when your hometown sports team gets into a championship tournament. There is electricity in the air, and every moment is filled with hope and eager anticipation. In this kind of climate, your body tingles with excitement over the news and surprises that come your way. Different parts of your body, including your arms, fingers, and legs, move as if you were dancing yourself through each day.

- You are completely focused and immersed in what you are doing. It is difficult for you to be distracted from what you are attending to, whether it be reading a book, performing your work, or enjoying a recreational activity. When you truly have passion for the task at hand, you fall naturally into it. This happens to mothers who enthusiastically bake a birthday cake, friends who travel to that special lake and throw out the fishing line, and adolescents who enthusiastically sing along with the radio.

- You are so absorbed in the flow of the moment that you give little time to dwelling on the past or future. Any glance backward or forward into time is done as if you were viewing an interesting movie. You relate to your life as a thrilling story, in which each new chapter is eagerly anticipated. When big life events happen to you—such as a wedding ceremony, the birth of a child, or getting a new job—you feel that your experiences are bigger than everyday life. In these moments you are more likely to notice that energy is moving through your body.

- You feel comfortably tired when it is time for you to enjoy a well-deserved rest. For instance, after a day's work in the garden you eagerly waited to plant, there's a good feeling of tiredness that comes upon you and helps you have a deep evening sleep. You know that it is natural to become tired, and accepting this and flowing with it contribute to revitalizing your life.

- Life in general feels natural, and it takes little effort to move vibrantly through the day. You really feel "on" and believe that it is likely that you will successfully meet every forthcoming challenge.
- Time often flies for you. Recall how the best novels and movies seem to end too quickly, no matter how long they are. Similarly, when your life is in tune, you can't seem to get enough time to do all that you want to do. Although you want to do many things, you still appreciate the occasional opportunity to do nothing at all.
- You often think about the importance of happiness and joy in your life, and you are not ashamed to allow yourself to have a good time. Perhaps you're ready at a moment's notice to take the family out for ice cream or to give a cheerful call to a good friend.
- You have high hopes about successfully realizing your greatest desires. What you desire for yourself also makes a positive contribution to others. There is no conflict between your personal success and your altruistic contributions. Your hopes breed success, and your success spreads the seeds of hope to your friends and family.
- Others see that you are filled with energy and vitality. Your energy flows forth when you are around them and they are vitalized by your presence. But while others may describe you as a dynamo, you have an intuition that this is not so much your energy as a resonant interaction that you are able to facilitate with others.
- It is difficult for you to get inappropriately irritated. You know that daily irritations, such as dripping faucets and rainy days, are the necessary spices that enrich the whole stew of life. If those moments take place when you can't avoid being irritated, you accept your own irritation and are not thrown off by it.
- You feel full of life and ready and eager to meet its challenges. You see all of life—its ups and downs, its episodes of health and illness, its abundance and scarcity—as helping make your life whole

and wholesome. You know that each day's imperfections are a necessary part of the big picture. This frees you to stop fighting life and to embrace fully what comes to you. You also know that making less resistance to the valleys of your life leads to higher climbs into the mountain peaks that are just around the bend.

- You celebrate with others when they show joy. Their joy is your joy, and because of this, people enjoy sharing their good news with you. As with a light, it doesn't matter who is holding the joy. It still illuminates the room for all who are present.

- You truly enjoy caring for your family, friends, and community. You have discovered that the quickest way to get the inner results you want is to act kindly and generously to those who live around you. Each day you wonder what you can do for someone else.

- You talk less about spirituality, but you walk in a spirited way. You are less interested in discussing your dreams than living them. You'd rather live with soul than hear about the latest academic understanding of what it means. For you there's more doing and less viewing of matters that refer to soul, spirit, and the sacred.

- You believe that life is filled with many treasures that await your finding them. When you wake up in the morning and hear a bird's song, you pay special attention and recognize the gift of that moment.

- Your life abounds with mystery. Every day is filled with wonder and enchantment, and you behold every sunset as a miracle. When your life is energized, it revitalizes your sense of magic and mystery. This is the most sacred mystery of all, and you find that many doors to uplifting experiences are opening to you.

These are the kinds of experiences that mark a tuned life. We may find ourselves automatically feeling this way during an energetic meeting at work where everyone's creative juices are flowing; during an inspired stroll through a museum; in our most passionate moments of making love; or when we are singing in a choir, hiking through a beautiful forest, helping a child learn to read, or being smitten with laughter during a free-flowing coversation with a close friend. The well-tuned life is richly graced with delightful sensations. I am not proposing that an energized person is always walking around with these feelings and states of mind. But when you are fully tuned, you will often find yourself touched by these kinds of experiences.

Our Bodies Are Instruments

We are delicate instruments, as sensitive as the finest strings on a Stradivarius violin, a Gibson guitar, or a Steinway grand piano. Don Campbell, the founder and director of the Institute for Music, Health, and Education in Boulder, Colorado, proposes that since the sounds we are capable of making come not only from our throat, but also from our solar plexus, the base of our spine, and the crown of our head, then our whole body—particularly the air column that the sound waves traverse—should be regarded as a vibrating string. Taking this perspective, I recommend that you regard yourself as a "body string" that requires regular tuning if you are to have a vibrant life. When we are in tune, we are prepared to resonate with life's vitality. When we are out of tune, nothing can help us revitalize ourselves except a retuning. It is a great miracle of life that in our most passionate moments, when we throw ourselves into what we are doing, we become automatically tuned and find ourselves feeling completely alive.

Have you ever become so lost in reading a great novel, playing your favorite sport, or watching a fascinating movie that you weren't aware of time moving forward? When this happens, you may forget to eat, miss outside stimuli, or even become unaware of your own body.

In this state of being perfectly tuned in to what you are doing, the vitalizing energy from life more easily flows through you.

There are Tibetan monks and Indian yogis who are known to be able to withstand the excruciating cold of the Himalayan Mountains without clothing, shelter, or any outside means of maintaining body warmth. Furthermore, some of these ascetic practitioners are capable of living on very little food. They are so perfectly in tune with their environment that they are able to be energized by the act of breathing.

These examples challenge the conventional view that we are simply a body machine. If we view the human being as a tuned instrument, there is no mystery involved in these amazing feats. The more tuned you are, the more able you are to have complete energy and vitality in whatever situation you happen to be in, from the peaks of the Himalayan Mountains to the hills and valleys of everyday life.

Consider the analogy of a Stradivarius violin. Even if you had the most valuable violin in the world, it would be worthless if it were played out of tune. Similarly, you are a miraculous creation of life, but the excellence, beauty, and creative expression that can come from you are not possible unless you, as an instrument, are tuned.

And, like the strings of a violin or a guitar, your body requires *constant* tuning. If you have ever attended a concert performance of a master guitarist, you may recall how often the strings were tuned. Any change encountered in the guitar's environment may throw the instrument off—a sudden blow to the instrument's body, the impact of inspired playing, or even a cold breeze blowing across the strings.

You, too, are vulnerable to the impacts, stresses, and changes that take place around you and in you. When you are walking down a sidewalk, completely absorbed in your thoughts, and you hear the blasting noise of a truck's horn or police siren, the shock of this unanticipated barrage of sound may suddenly throw you out of tune. You subsequently feel disoriented or dizzy and are bewildered to find that it feels as if energy has been drained out of you.

The same thing may happen when you lose your temper and succumb to the inner and outer flow of anger. This burst of hot emotion typically leaves you feeling exhausted, making you vulnerable to getting sick. When I taught family therapy in various university clinics, I was amazed to see how often blowups in interpersonal relations were followed by someone getting a cold or the flu, or the onset of another symptom. I am not saying that getting angry always makes you sick, but an out-of-control emotional bout does wreck whatever state of tuning you held before you went into the fit, leaving you with less life energy and thereby making you more vulnerable to disease.

It doesn't take an emotional outburst or a jarring experience to throw you off. The simple trials and tribulations of each day can pull you out of tune. When you slip into binge worrying, get nervous about your work, get too competitive, push yourself too hard, or forget to take a deep breath and pause to notice the world that surrounds you, it is likely that you will begin to go out of tune.

You need to be able to recognize the kinds of experiences that tend to throw you out of tune and know when to take a momentary break from your daily activities to bring yourself back into a tuned state of being. This is how you begin moving toward energizing your life.

Being Tuned Is an Experience in Absorption

The way the great novelist Aldous Huxley wrote his books is a wonderful example of being powerfully tuned. As Huxley described it to the American hypnotist Milton H. Erickson, he would enter into a deeply reflective state that enabled him to mentally set aside anything not pertinent to his writing.* He was so completely focused that he could perform physical acts without any conscious awareness. For instance, one afternoon while he was deeply engaged in writing, the mailman rang the doorbell. Huxley walked to the door, opened it, took a special delivery letter, immediately closed the door, put the letter on a table, and then walked to his chair and continued his work. When his wife came home and discovered the letter, he had absolutely no conscious recollection that it had arrived.

This same state of complete absorption was behind the so-called "absentmindedness" of Norbert Wiener, the mathematical genius and MIT professor who invented the science of cybernetics. Several of his former students told me that Professor Wiener would become so absorbed in his thoughts about mathematics that he would have to hold out a finger to trace the edge of the hallway so that he could walk while thinking or reading. One day he walked down a corridor at MIT in this way, carefully rubbing his finger along the wall. Oblivious of the fact that he was coming to the open door of a classroom, he proceeded to walk into the room and walk around it, with no idea that he was doing so, in the midst of a class meeting. Then out and on he went, until he arrived safely at his office. Like Huxley, Wiener could become so absorbed in his work that he was not distracted by anything, yet he was under the complete guidance and protection offered by unconscious aspects of his being.

Have you ever driven your car and found that all of a sudden you are so absorbed in your thoughts that you are completely zoned out, with no conscious awareness of your driving? When you come back to an awareness of being in the car, you are startled because you recog-

---

*See *The Collected Papers of Milton H. Erickson on Hypnosis*, vol. I, Ernest Rossi, ed. New York: Irvington, 1980.

nize that you were not conscious of the previous seconds or minutes. Even though you can't remember driving the car in such circumstances, you know that you obviously did so in some unconscious form of autopilot.

Throughout our everyday life we are familiar with these episodes of complete absorption, but we typically excuse them as a momentary "mental lapse." What we overlook is that these states of complete absorption bring us into a tuned state of being. When you step out of such a state, you feel energized and revitalized. What happens to you in this state? The answer is both simple and profound.

The Rhythm of the Earth

Physicists have found that the earth resonates at around 7.83 cycles per second. This is the measurement of the magnetic wave frequencies that pulse between the earth's surface and the ionosphere, the part of the atmosphere that begins at about twenty-five miles above the earth. Scientists refer to this rhythm as the Schumann resonance and have proposed that it is the pulse or heartbeat of earth itself. Thus, the ocean of universal life force that we live in has a pulse, a natural rhythm, just like the waves and tides in the world's oceans.

Our bodies are able to move with this very same rhythm. In fact, when we are in a deep state of absorption, our brain waves pulse at 7.83 beats per second: this is called the alpha frequency. What happens when we resonate with this rhythm is that we fall into the same beat as the universal life force, enabling a flow of energy from the ocean of energy that surrounds us directly into the body. The natural way to open the gate that lets in the universal life force is to simply resonate with life's natural pulse. When we fall into this rhythm, we feel completely absorbed and tuned as the energy naturally flows through us.

To help explain how this can take place, consider the following physical experiment. Take two tuned violins and place one of them on a table while playing a note on the other one. If you carefully observe both these instruments, you will find that the same string being played on one violin is also being hummed on the violin that rests on the table. In this *sympathetic resonance* between the two violins, the acoustical energy created by the first violin is actually transferred to the second violin.

The energy from one vibrating string is able to be transferred to another string when it is harmonically tuned to the other's frequency. When any two systems are harmonically tuned, they are said to be resonant with one another, and this is what enables energy in one system to be transferred to another. When we tune ourselves to be in harmony with the universal life force, its energy is readily transferred to us, in the same way that the sound of one vibrating violin string is able to energize and sound a tuned string of another instrument.

Being in Tune with Each Other

As a family therapist I have observed mothers and fathers who were so in tune with their children that they could feel the child's sensory experience. If the child's finger was cut, the parent would actually feel the same pain. Sometimes these parents were so overtuned to their child that their experiences became too enmeshed. Parent and child would finish sentences for each other and sometimes have the same dreams. This kind of tuning has also been expressed in the lives of identical twins who are extraordinarily close to one another. It's been observed that you can bump into one twin and find that the other twin says "Ouch!"

Closer to everyday experience are those special moments when we find ourselves falling into natural attunement with another person, whether it be in dance, basketball, conversation, or intimate kissing. When you are in perfect tune with another person, your experience is simultaneously realized by the other, creating an incredible possibility for unified movement and expression. This is the experience of complete absorption that often carries you into a tuned state of being. You also may be in tune with other realms of experience that don't necessarily involve the participation of another human being. For example, you can become in perfect tune with music you are hearing, or with a book you are reading, a landscape you are beholding, or a breeze that you feel blowing across your face. When you're in tune with whatever you happen to encounter, the pulse of the other can move you into an energetic resonance with it.

In the laboratory, scientists have found that when two wave patterns of identical frequency and amplitude meet one another, they can produce a waveform that is twice the height of the original waveform. In other words, this builds up the amplitude or volume of the sound. When we resonate with the universal life force, we too build up the energy within us. It becomes amplified, and we feel reenergized and revitalized. When audience members clap their hands together in the same pulse, it sounds like a singular powerful hand clap. Similarly, when we move in rhythm with the pulse of music, whether it be through dance or simply tapping our toes, we experience the beat more powerfully. The popular notion of a soul mate or soul friend carries the truth that we are strongly drawn to certain people because their frequencies bring forth a natural resonance that is mutually energizing.

On the other hand, when two waves meet that are opposing patterns, the result is that they cancel each other out. When two dancers are really out of sync with one another, they can easily trip and fall to the floor. Similarly, when a musical group is not in rhythm, the music will not be able to move forward—the flow will fall apart and simply stop. This is called *destructive interference.* The implication for us in our everyday life is that if we vibrate at a frequency that is out of sync with that of the universal life force, we will feel a cancellation and loss of our vitality and find that our energy is being drained away. In this view, being tired is essentially a condition of being out of sync with the universal life force.

Of course it is not always as simple as two frequencies either amplifying each other or canceling each other out. Sometimes we interact with other frequencies and create a more complex harmonic pattern, something that isn't simply an amplification or a cancellation. Overall, however, we still find it useful to differentiate between those interactions that tend to amplify our energy and those that tend to drain us. Other interactions are somewhere in between, in the middle ground of diverse harmonic patterns, some more energizing than others.

Finding Our Own Frequencies
The research of Dr. Valerie V. Hunt, a physiologist at the University of California at Los Angeles, indicates that the human body is an electromagnetic field with frequencies that can be measured in a laboratory. Her work suggests that each of us came into this world with a frequency (or set of frequencies) that is ideal for us. When we resonate at that particular frequency, we experience an optimal state of health and well-being and find ourselves to be at our peak performance. The natural frequency of each human being is capable of entering into a harmonic relationship with the universal life force. These sympathetic resonances with life's pulse provide a natural bridge for you to enter into its endless supply of energy.

Although we all have different frequencies, this does not mean that some of us are destined to have more or less life energy than others. If my natural frequency is lower than yours, this does not mean that you will have higher energy than I do. It only means that the best way for me to have a sympathetic resonance with the life force is to do so through the low frequency that is most natural for me. Each person's natural frequency is simply the pulse which, for that person, is the surest and purest route to making connection with the life force.

For the sake of illustration, let us assume that the frequency of the life force is the same as the musical note that is called "middle C" on the piano keyboard. The natural frequencies that are available to us could then be said to be those notes that are in natural harmony with middle C. For instance, you might naturally resonate as a G or as an E, either of which is in simple harmony with C. What is important is that your frequency be in a harmonic relationship with the frequency of life.

Lower frequencies are associated with the activities of the physical body. This may involve sports, dance, large body movements, or the fine motor skills of one's fingers. If you resonate well with low frequencies, then a career in sports or one involving challenging physical movements is worth exploring. A midrange frequency indicates a natural bent for intellectual forms of activity, whereas higher frequencies correspond with intuitive ways of knowing. The highest frequencies enter the realms of spirituality that range from creative and artistic talents to healing others and, finally, to mystical experiences.

When you are most resonant with your natural frequency, you are healthiest and are best promoting your own state of well-being. I would venture to guess that Michael Jordan is most likely to get himself tuned while throwing himself into a basketball game, whereas Stephen Hawking will get tuned while pursuing an abstract scientific theory and the Dalai Lama is more likely to be finely tuned as he pursues a deep contemplative practice. Jordan is at a natural low frequency; it makes little sense for him to tune himself through literary writing and more sense for him to fall into the poetry of athletic motion. Likewise, why would the Dalai Lama play basketball to get himself tuned? He functions at a natural high frequency—a tenor of life, we could say—and that is the surest path for him to find his tuning and vitality.

Your natural frequency will often have a particular physical feeling associated with it. When people are vibrating at their natural beat, they sometimes feel a certain "buzz," have a tingly feeling in the gut, experience a pleasant sensation of light-headedness, or feel a rhythmic pulse surge through the chest. Typically, people who resonate most naturally with low frequencies feel it in the belly or solar plexus, whereas midrange frequencies play themselves out in the chest and heart region, and high frequencies tend to be felt in the head.

Each person is equipped with physical, emotional, intellectual, healing, and spiritual tools for an entire life span. However, our most natural frequency emphasizes the specific areas in which we are most naturally inclined to succeed. Knowing your frequency may be a more powerful insight than knowing any psychological, medical, or astrological assessment, because it leads you to the kind of life that will be more likely to bring the universal life force into you.

A Simple Self-Test to Help You Find Your Natural Frequency

What is your frequency? You can easily determine whether you are more naturally inclined toward a low, medium, or high frequency by asking yourself some simple questions. All of these questions address whether you are more naturally drawn to physical, intellectual, or intuitive pursuits. Here's a quick self-test to help you find your frequency:

1. What do you most identify with?
   ____ body   ____ mind   ____ soul
2. What activity was most natural to you in school?
   ____ sports   ____ academic work
   ____ creative and imaginative pursuits
3. Which would you rather have?
   ____ great body   ____ high IQ   ____ creativity
4. What are you most impressed with?
   ____ world championship in a sport
   ____ Nobel Prize in physics
   ____ Pulitzer Prize for poetry
5. What would you rather be able to do?
   ____ run a mile
   ____ solve a challenging mathematical problem
   ____ create a work of art
6. Which experience would you enjoy most?
   ____ dancing   ____ reading a book
   ____ entering a meditative state
7. Which of these attributes do you value most?
   ____ being physically fit
   ____ being skilled in reason and logic
   ____ having natural intuition

After answering these questions, look to see whether you tended to give the first, second, or third answer. If you favored the first answer, you are probably more inclined toward a low frequency, whereas the second answer suggests a midrange frequency and the third implies a natural inclination toward higher frequencies. Keep in mind that higher frequencies are not better than lower ones, any more than a higher-pitched sound is better than a low tone. Knowing your frequency is similar to finding out whether your voice is more suited for being a bass, a baritone-alto, or a tenor-soprano. Your frequency simply represents the most natural vibration of your body string. It is easiest for you to sound this frequency and to use it to enter into resonances that can tune your whole being.

It follows that it is important for you to do the kind of activities that are most related to your natural frequency. If you are a low-frequency person, then make certain that your life is filled with physical activity or exercise. For example, I have seen low-frequency people who were tired and believed that they suffered from depression but were not involved in any physical exercise. Getting them to move with physical exercise and activity made a dramatic difference in their state of being and helped bring them back into their naturally tuned frequency. Similarly, high-frequency people who do not provide time for contemplative work and creative expression can become quite agitated, irritable, and restless—in other words, out of tune. Helping get them back on track is often as easy as scheduling an hour to pursue a high-frequency activity, such as creating a poem, a song, or a painting.

Rather than search for a sophisticated scientific measurement of your frequency spectrum, I suggest that you draw upon some common sense. When you feel vibrant and energetically alive, examine the kind of activity and relationships you are in. If it's a certain kind of physical activity, motion, mental exercise, emotional state, or way of contemplating, see it as representing the frequency of activity that is easy for you to enter. It is a sign of your natural frequency. The more grounded the experience—that is, the more rooted to physical activity—the lower the frequency. The more you enter the mental, intuitive, and nonmaterial realms, the higher the frequency.

Energy Fingerprints

Although you may find that you now seem to be more inclined to low, medium, or high frequencies, you should realize that there are other openings and resonances you can learn that will take you across the entire spectrum of life. As noted above, scientists such as Dr. Valerie Hunter have physically measured the vibrations and frequencies of people's energy fields. Hunter's research, over a period of more than twenty years, has found that each person has a unique energy field characterized not only by its frequency and power (amplitude), but also by the way the energy is impeded or unimpeded in its flow through particular body areas. These *energy fingerprints* reveal the complexity of your energy field, which determines how many different kinds of resonant interactions you can, at present, enter into. A narrow vibrational spectrum means that you are limited in the ways you can positively resonate with the world. For instance, if you are "turned on" and tuned only by physical activity, you have a limited range of ways in which you can be energized by life. If this is the case, you have yet to discover the whole world of intellectual, intuitive, and creative offerings. On the other hand, a wide spectrum assures you of more opportunities for energetic interactions in the course of each day. Here you are more open to the many different kinds of experiences that life presents. For example, a well-known publishing executive sometimes feels energized and powerfully alive when she's competing on her horse, but at other times she finds herself maximally vibrant when absorbed in an editorial discussion. Her energy fingerprint indicates both physical and intellectual frequencies.

Clearly, the complete mapping of our energy processes is complex. Although it is true that we each tend to vibrate more naturally in certain frequencies, this is not the whole picture. You change throughout the day as well as through the various stages of your life. Although you may want to be aware of the frequencies which are most natural for you and those with which you are having difficulties, do not take these generalizations too rigidly. At any moment you may become opened to a different frequency through an interaction that takes you to a new vibrational experience.

For instance, when you have a new experience, like dancing for the first time, you open yourself to a pulse or rhythm you haven't felt before. When this pulse is integrated into your body, it is capable of changing the range and quality of your energetic relations with others. This is how dance and rhythm provide a powerful agent of change.

The more you learn to enter into more interactional resonances that energize you, the more your daily life will be charged and revitalized. As you will later see, the way to expand your repertoire of resonances is found in the practice of Autokinetics. Its natural motions will introduce you to new frequencies and vibrational states. With it, you will learn to expand the possibilities for bringing forth new energetic interactions in your daily life.

Stay Tuned

When you are truly tuned to the pulse of life, you find that you no longer have to exercise strong willpower and discipline to accomplish what you desire. Life begins to happen naturally, without much effort, and sometimes the movement of your life is so smooth that you feel as if you are just going along for the ride. This effortless living is the surest sign that the life force is with you. Like a river that flows naturally down its banks, your life moves without any resistance or interruption. Nothing can get to you, no matter how challenging the situation happens to be, as long as you are filled with the universal life force.

The reason that you get too tired is that you are fighting life or trying to force it to work for you. Any resistance to life is friction that brings you out of tune and results in your feeling depleted and tired. The trick to life is finding and then committing yourself to doing what you truly enjoy, what is most natural for you. If you are doing something because you think you should, perhaps because your parents or early schoolteachers put it into your mind that this was what you were supposed to do with your life, then you may be in trouble. You can't optimize the quality of your life by forcing yourself to do what is unnatural. If you weren't meant to be a lawyer and you have a body that calls for physical activity, then consider moving yourself to a lower frequency. On the other hand, if your body can't keep up with the activities that your job demands, look for a desk job that pulses more naturally with your preferred frequency.

Overcontrolling your life is another way of fighting the natural call of life. You resist what you think you don't want and pull in what you think you desire. This is what makes you so tired. But if you enter the stream that was meant to carry your life, there need be no resisting or pulling—only natural movement.

There is a way of feeling tired that is natural. It is the desire of the body to stop and take a rest. This tiredness doesn't have to be resisted but can be accepted and used to direct your retuning. Fighting your tired state is not natural. Any combat against your tiredness will further wear you down and lead you to the affliction of our time—the never-ending struggle against fatigue. You must learn to flow in and out of your everyday tiredness so that it contributes to the rhythms that tune you to the universal life force. In other words, the transition between feeling tired and feeling energized is a natural movement that must be accepted and worked with if you want to revitalize your life.

Your *body* is the instrument of your life. It is the responsibility of your *mind* to be in charge of tuning this instrument. Your mind should, this very moment, pledge to accept its principal role as the tuner of your body. It has no business venturing too far away from this purpose. It should take care of its primary business: seeing to it that your instrument is kept tuned.

When your body is cared for and tuned by your mind, it is ready and available for your *soul* to express its creative desires. In this interwoven, holistic connection of your body, mind, and soul, it is your soul that plays the music of your life. When your mind tunes your body, your soul is called upon to play the instrument of your life, making your everyday presence a beautiful and inspiring contribution.

You fall into unnatural tiredness when your soul is absent and your mind tries to force some music from a weary, out-of-tune instrument. I assure you that if you mindfully attend to the tuning of your body instrument, its readiness to make music will call forth your soul to creatively express your life upon it.

It is now time for you to learn how to tune yourself to life and discover how you may bring in its revitalizing energy. As you will soon discover, the secret of a successful energy break involves the act of moving your body to be resonant with the pulse of life itself.

CHAPTER TWO

The Three-Step Technique

■——————————————————

If you go into a classroom of children you will see that no matter what the teacher says to them, they will not sit still. Children are naturally impelled to move their bodies. If they are sitting in a chair, you may see their legs and bodies swinging and swaying to a natural rhythm. Perhaps you can recall how you once sat in the classroom with your legs crossed while one leg and foot bounced in a steady rhythm, or how your body rocked forward and backward in a hypnotic pulse as the teacher talked about some subject that just didn't quite grab your attention. Or maybe your fingertips always had to drum the top of your desk, or both of your feet bounced on the floor as if they were attached to springs.

These movements easily took us into daydreams and trancelike states and were not encouraged by our teachers and caretakers. Like today's children, we were told to be still, to stop being so fidgety, and to settle down. I remember a friend of mine always being asked by our grade school teacher, "Randy, do you have ants in your pants?"

As children our bodies had an innate wisdom that moved us to fall into the natural rhythms that brought us into harmony with the life force around us. We kept ourselves energized, much to the frustration of our parents and teachers, by these simple vibratory movements, though we had no idea that this was what we were doing. What happened along the way was that we were instructed to sit still and stop making these spontaneous movements. Quite literally, the free-flowing motions were taken away from us. By the time we reached high school and college we no longer rocked in our chairs, and many of us found that we had little life force during a teacher's lecture. It took great effort to stay alert and awake in school until we could get out of class and allow our bodies to move freely in the hallways.

Child rearing is radically different on the South Pacific island of Bali. There, adults encourage their children to make natural movements. The anthropologists Margaret Mead and Gregory Bateson discovered that Balinese parents teach their children how to lift the leg in a certain way that precipitates an oscillating movement called a muscle "clonus." This is an experience that we all know, and it is easily produced: While sitting with your feet on the floor, move one foot back until your heel is off the floor, with the ball of your foot supporting the weight of your leg. At the right angle, an oscillation will start in that calf muscle, with a frequency of about eight cycles per second.

In Bali, children are taught to bring forth these automatic muscle oscillations and use them to trigger a trance state. In this way they may automatically dance themselves through the activities of each day, vitalizing themselves with their natural movements.

As a child, you, too, created these natural movements and, without knowing it, entered into energizing trance states. I want to take you back to the natural movements and rhythms that you once had as a child and return them to your daily life. These movements were the body's automatic way of energizing itself. Your task is to become familiar with how you can use these movements and rhythms as a natural way of moving yourself into the pulse of the universal life force.

Moving from Ancient Ways to a Contemporary Practice

In the practice of *seiki-jutsu*, the Japanese art of (*jutsu*) working with the life force (*seiki*) that I describe in Chapter Five, you are asked to sit on a wooden bench and then encourage your body to fall into any simple movement. You may sway from side to side, back and forth, or in circular or elliptical patterns, or bob up and down. The movement may be more in your neck, at the base of your spine, or in your arms or legs. As you sit on the bench and allow your body to move, it is permissible to fall into any imaginable motion. The pattern may stay locked in one form, or it may change often. In *seiki-jutsu*, your body is allowed to play with these motions, and in doing this you learn to fall into a motion so natural that you feel that you aren't making it but it is moving you.

In other words, *seiki-jutsu* takes you back to the time when you were a child and you allowed your body to make natural movements. In that space there was no right or wrong movement, no conscious choreography. Now as an adult you are to return to those freely expressed movements and aim for an outcome that you probably were not conscious of as a child. Now you will knowingly use this freedom of expression to take you into an automatic movement, one that takes place without your having to make it happen. This is the "tuning zone," the place of complete absorption, and when you fall into its dreamy, trancelike state, you must learn to ride it out, allowing it to tune you in a natural way. Here you enter into a sympathetic resonance with the universal life force and find that it energizes and revitalizes your whole being.

In my travels around the world, I have found that many cultures go through elaborate rituals and ordeals in order to get their people to fall into these natural motions and rhythms. Sometimes this involves dancing all night, and at other times it involves having an energized shaman pulse rhythms into their bodies. In *seiki-jutsu,* it is assumed that you must first be "filled with *seiki.*" In the traditional scenario, you develop a close relationship with a master practitioner and become increasingly comfortable with his or her hands-on work. As your body learns to trust and fully accept the energized hands of the master, you eventually are taken to a special place where it is believed that the earth's energy is strong, and there a ceremonial event takes place. The *seiki* master stirs up the life force and then brings it into your body in a powerful way. Following this "transmission of *seiki,*" as it is called, your body tends to naturally enter into gentle rocking motions. This is taken as a sign that you have received *seiki,* and from that moment on you are told to initiate the practice of rocking or spontaneously moving on a daily basis.

I have found that it is not necessary for you to be filled with the universal life energy in this dramatic way as a prerequisite for initiating the energizing movements. Anyone at any time can start moving into these natural rhythms. Children do it, and even animals do it. Have you ever watched a dog or cat take a stretch or have a super-yawn? The whole body stretches out, and then at the final moment the animal vibrates and shakes. This is one of the ways animals naturally tune themselves. Try it yourself. The next time you feel a big yawn coming on, go for it and allow that yawn to become a super-yawn. At the end of the yawn, when your mouth is open as wide as it can possibly get, allow your body to vibrate and shake. If you get fully into this, you'll find out what's going on with the household pet. You'll find a natural way of helping yourself move into a tuned state.

Autokinetics

"Kinetics" is defined by *Webster's International Dictionary* as "relating to the motion of material bodies and the forces and energy associated therewith." Automatic kinetics, or *Autokinetics* for short, is therefore the practice of making automatic or spontaneous body movements that bring forth life energy. There are three simple steps that constitute the practice of Autokinetics. However, unlike aerobic exercise, yoga, diets, and innumerable other therapeutic programs, Autokinetics does not require any willpower, discipline, or stamina.

Some people hesitate to try out anything new because they remember all the work it took with previous health programs, strategies, and techniques. What I offer you differs from anything else you have ever tried because it involves *no work.* I am inviting you to have a true energy break, a recess time when you practice some effortless, playful movement. When you become a master of this energizing recess, endless benefits will flow into your life. Again, Autokinetics does not ask you to force any movement, thought, belief, understanding, attitude, or feeling. It only asks that you take a ten-minute break to allow yourself to move as your body desires, doing so without purpose, without work, and without effort. In this break from the manic demands of everyday life, life's energy will come to you, free of any financial charge, but ready to energetically charge your whole being.

Don't worry if you are a little timid about taking the first step. Know that others have felt the same inhibitions and trepidation, but they went on to give Autokinetics a try. Although the explanations may sound a bit wordy at first, when you actually try the three steps you will find that Autokinetics is quickly learned. Imagine trying to read a book that teaches you how to ride a bicycle. It might seem complicated until you simply got on the bike and tried to ride. As you now know, once you get the hang of it, riding a bicycle falls into place and seems completely natural. You are then able to do it with ease for the rest of your life. This is even more true for Autokinetics. Once you feel the natural motion your body is already programmed to deliver, you won't be able to live without it. There won't be a single day that goes by without an energy break. These movements will help you find the peace, success, and bliss you desire.

The Three-Step Technique

When we strip away the cultural ornamentation, mythological beliefs, and historical customs, we find that all of the world's most powerful healing practices are about getting your body to be in tune with the universal life force. The easiest entry into this tuning process is to get your body to pulse with life's beat, thereby creating the kind of positive resonance that transfers life energy into you.

I have identified and simplified the core of the ancient healing and revitalizing practices, paring them down to their essential principles, so that they may be easily learned and practiced by anyone without having to receive extensive training or religious indoctrination. These principles, which constitute the practice of Autokinetics, reduce themselves to three easy steps that are outlined for you as follows:

- *Step one. Initiate the body rhythm.* Sit and start a rocking motion of your body that turns into a natural, spontaneous rhythm.
- *Step two. Improvise movement.* Let yourself engage in improvised body expression, ranging from small movements to dance-like postures and gestures, and be open to making impromptu sounds.
- *Step three. Enter the tuning zone.* Allow this free and spontaneous expression of your body to carry you into the hypnotic experience of the "tuning zone."

Now let's examine each of these steps and carry you to the easiest and most natural way you can have an energy break.

Step One: Initiate the Body Rhythm

Find yourself a bench, stool, or chair to use for this practice. The Japanese tradition of *seiki-jutsu* uses a wooden bench that is 17 inches high, with a seat measuring 16 by 9 inches. However, it doesn't matter what kind of chair you use as long as you are able to move your whole body easily while sitting on it. You do not want to sit in a chair that you readily sink or fall back into. A flat surface is best, and soft, deep cushions or plush upholstery should be avoided.

When you sit down to start this practice, take a deep breath, close your eyes, and take a moment to calm and slow down your mind. Then press the inner corner of each eyeball with the middle or second finger of each hand, as shown in Figure 1. This sends a signal to your autonomic nervous system that you are beginning the practice of Autokinetics.

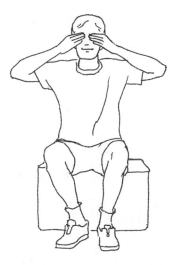

At this point, your goal is to initiate a rocking motion of your body. In the beginning you can purposefully cause this movement yourself, never worrying whether you are making the right motion or not. *In this practice there are no right or wrong movements.* You may start with a rocking movement of your lower back, or you may want to focus on a rocking motion of your head. In the beginning you are simply getting a motion started that will eventually fall into an automatic movement that happens without any conscious effort on your part. As you move your body, keep in mind the words of Albert Einstein: "Nothing happens until something moves."

This first step is analogous to tuning a guitar string. You need to tighten and loosen the string many times by turning the tuning key (a metal rod that the string is attached to) back and forth in order to get it just right. As you move your body instrument in any direction—back and forth, side to side, or in circular patterns—do not be concerned with how slow or fast you are; just allow movement to take place. Sometimes it is helpful to think of yourself as a toy top that has been wound up through the activities, feelings, and thoughts of the previous hours or days. When you sit down to do this practice, you allow that wound-up tension to be released; and in so doing, your body begins to literally unwind, manifesting this release as a rocking, vibrating, coiling motion.

In the beginning, it may take a minute or two for you to get an appropriate start-off motion. As you become more acquainted with the technique, the first step will take less than a minute, and it may require only a few seconds for you to get the motions initiated in the right way.

I worked with a retired pilot from Nevada who had plenty of time to spend with his three grandchildren. Accordingly, he wanted to have as much energy as possible so he could fully relish every special moment with them. He began his energy break as if he were getting ready to fly a small propeller-driven airplane. When he sat in his chair to start his practice, his right hand and arm would move forward as if he were turning on a switch to start the plane's engine. As he did this, he imagined hearing the sound of a propeller starting to turn. He then began making a circular movement of his upper torso, allowing it to settle into a natural vibration and then take him into what was usually an imaginary flight. This was how he started his practice of Autokinetics and brought forth a personal energy break—by literally turning on an imaginary switch to initiate its movement.

The transition from *making* body movements to falling into a *natural rhythm* that seems to be made independent of your efforts is the key moment in Autokinetics. It doesn't matter what you do to make this transition. Since everyone will find his or her own path into it, and it can be different each time you do it, do not worry about whether you are doing it right. With this in mind you may be better off trying to make a "wrong" movement, because what your mind thinks is wrong may trip your body out of the control of your habitual mind, allowing you to fall into the flow of a naturally moving rhythm. You will know it when you fall into the natural rhythm, even if it lasts only a few minutes or seconds.

Here are some of the tricks I have suggested that people try in order to trigger a natural body rhythm:

Batter Up!   One way of thinking about this first step is to see it as a time for "getting ready." When you watch a major league baseball game, you notice that each batter goes through a whole series of motions before he hits the ball. These movements are all about getting ready to step into the batter's box and take a swing. In fact, as a batter prepares to step up to home plate and take a swing, you see rituals that are every bit as complex, elaborate, and superstitious as the cere-monies of ancient tribal people. The head and torso are swung left and right, arms and hands are wiggled, the rear end is shaken, and unique body gestures and movements are made. And then the batter steps up to the plate and lets his mind forget about making anything happen. If he's truly ready, he doesn't have to think about hitting: it will take place spontaneously and effortlessly. If he thinks too much about hit-ting the ball, it will disturb his natural groove and throw him out of sync with the movements required to get a hit.

The same is true for Autokinetics. You must first do some move-ments that simply get you ready to move into the effortless motions of tuning yourself. You can experiment with your own personalized body ritual, much like that of a professional baseball hitter, so that you can enter into some naturally occurring body movements. Use this ritual as a way of tricking yourself into falling into a natural rhythm—the whole purpose of the first step of this practice.

The "Body Shake" I sometimes recommend that people try to be completely spastic for a minute, vigorously mobilizing all the parts of the body that they can move. Wiggle your toes and fingers, shake your arms and legs, twist your waist, bounce up and down, twist your head from side to side, huff and puff so as to move your chest, and so forth. When you max out or hit the peak with these movements, come to an immediate stop and encourage your body to fall into the most natural movement it can realize.

I recommend the "body shake" because it tends to get the life force buzzing in your body, and its wild movements distract your mind from tracking what you are doing, thus freeing you from being con-trolled by your thought processes. When you shake yourself and suddenly stop, you are hoping that you accidentally fall into a natural rhythmic movement. Allow this movement to be small—a subtle and gentle rocking of the head or whole body. The key here is that you *feel* a natural rhythm in your body. Pay no attention to what it may look like; just focus on the unique feeling of being in free, natural, rhythmic motion.

Imitating the Natural Movement of a Pendulum Another trick that may help you fall into a natural rhythm involves getting yourself a pendulum. You can purchase one or make one yourself. One easy way to make one is to go to a sporting goods store that sells fishing supplies and purchase a small lead weight. Simply tie some thread, fishing line, or string to it, and you have yourself a fine pendulum. The next time you sit to take an energy break, bring your pendulum and hold it in front of you with one hand. Experiment with holding it in different places—above your head, in front of your chest, below your knees, and so forth. Notice how easy it is for the pendulum to fall into a state where it moves on its own. It may rock back and forth or sway from side to side or move in circular orbits.

According to some superstitious beliefs, these automatic movements of the pendulum are made by "spirits," since the person holding it is often surprised by the way it seems to move on its own, changing its motion as if it were alive. According to other beliefs, it is moved by the natural energies of the earth and can therefore be used to dowse for water or precious metals.

In fact, the pendulum is moved by the pulse of your own field of energy. This energy may make resonant interactions with the earth, but it indicates *your* movement, not those of any extraneous entity or outside force, so using a pendulum is an easy way to introduce yourself to the natural movements you are trying to more fully embrace. As you hold this pendulum in front of you, focus all of your mind on tracking its motion. Memorize its pattern of movement and then close your eyes and let your body move in the same pattern, as if you were now the pendulum. Imagine that you are being held by a string and that your whole body is actually suspended by it, so that your body could swing in the same way as the pendulum you hold. Again, allow the motion to be small if that is how it naturally comes forth, and do not be concerned with any display of huge, obvious movements. Allow the smallest movements to grow larger if they do so naturally, or allow them to get smaller if that's how you are pulled.

When I introduce people to the swinging motion of a pendulum, I remind them of the old days of hypnosis, when the hypnotist would swing a pendulum in front of the subject's eyes and suggest that its movement would bring on a trance. One of my clients was a legal secretary and the single parent of two small children. She wanted a practice that would not only give her more energy, but also relax her from the manic workload she was carrying. I suggested that she think about the pendulum as something that could hypnotize her whole body when she allowed her body to move with it. In this trance, her body movements would easily and deeply progress into all the steps of Autokinetics, doing so with a completely natural rhythm that proved to be an effective energy break for her.

Moving with the Wind   I have suggested that clients listen to recordings of the wind blowing, something you can purchase in the special effects section of any large CD and tape store. I recommend that they imagine themselves as a tree. As they hear the sounds of the wind blowing, they move with it as if they were that imaginary tree. This also can be practiced standing up outdoors on a windy day, so that you join ranks with the other moving trees and move with them as the wind blows. This is one of the oldest ways of teaching natural movement, and it is as effective a teaching image and practice today as it was thousands of years ago in China.

One of my clients, a young sushi chef in New York, went to Central Park on a windy spring afternoon and tried this practice of natural movement. He found that doing it once was enough for his body to incorporate the natural movements that a tree in a breeze can make. He still uses his memory of moving like a tree as a way to help start the natural motions required with Autokinetics.

The Rocking Chair Primer If you feel somewhat inhibited or are not comfortable with making a lot of external motion, then a rocking chair may be the best place for you to begin. Find a rocking chair that is easy to rock. Do your Autokinetics in this chair, experimenting with various rocking motions until you are able to fall into a small movement that seems to be taking place independent of you. When this happens you will feel like the chair is rocking itself and that you have nothing to do with its movement. As simple as this method may seem, this is one of the most powerful means of learning to initiate an automatic movement. I personally used this method when I began working with Autokinetics.

I want to make it clear that it is not always necessary for you to begin Autokinetics by engaging in any of these suggested procedures. These are mentioned as examples of how you might trick or trip yourself into the experience of a natural movement. Once you've had an experience or two with feeling your body move naturally, you will learn how to go into such movement with little preparation. But in the beginning, you may have to explore various ways of awakening to this motion—of bringing it into your awareness. You are already wired to have this experience in your daily life. You now have to find a way to turn it on.

To summarize step one: you may try anything that helps you fall into a natural rhythmic movement, whether it involves swinging with a pendulum, shaking your body to be loose, swaying with the wind, or rocking in a way that helps free you from your conscious mind. You may also sit down on your practice seat and simply wait for the rhythm to come forth. Give yourself an evening, if you wish, to tinker with all the motions you can make, knowing that there is no right or wrong movement. In trying a wide variety of motions, you hope for the kind of accident that will trip you into a natural movement.

This step will be the most important one in your beginning work with Autokinetics, and you should therefore take as much time as necessary for you to get a natural rhythm. Sometimes you may spend most of the time trying to get this rhythm going, or find yourself falling in and out of it. This is natural, and you should be patient with your learning. It bears repeating that over time, this step will take only a few seconds or a minute at most to complete. Once your body is familiar with doing this, it will take place almost automatically.

In his classic book *Zen in the Art of Archery,* Eugen Herrigel writes of living in Japan and learning the art of archery from a Zen master. Over and over, his master would proclaim: "The right art is purposeless, aimless! The more obstinately you try to learn how to shoot the arrow for the sake of hitting the goal, the less you will succeed in the one and the further the other will recede." Similarly, the more you try purposefully to get a natural rhythm, the further from success you may drift. The challenge for you is to tinker and play with as many movements as you can, and then wait patiently.

This patience of waiting for the accident that trips you into the natural rhythm is poetically described by Herrigel's Zen master:

It is all so simple. You can learn from an ordinary bamboo leaf what ought to happen. It bends lower and lower under the weight of snow. Suddenly the snow slips to the ground without the leaf having stirred.

In this natural state of affairs, a whole pattern rather than a spurt of conscious will or purposeful intention triggers the action. As you find yourself falling into the natural rhythm, you will find that it comes of its own accord, without being forced. You stop swimming against the current. No longer do you merely react to anything, and you do not force a movement. You become as flexible as a bamboo leaf that yields to the weight of snow or the movement of wind, not because you are passive but because you've become free, loose, and springy, able to move with the natural currents that flow through.

Step Two: Improvise Movement

When your actions are effortless and you find yourself surprised by the ease at which they come forth, you will find that you have truly entered a spontaneous way of being. In this state of flow you are *improvising*—that is, making your own movements as you go along, as opposed to rigidly following some template or static recipe for action.

Ken Werner, one of the premier jazz musicians of our time, gave a lecture at the International Association of Jazz Educators in 1991 and described his experience of improvising: "The music is there already before you play it. . . . All you have to do is tap into it and it's going to flow out at such an alarming rate that the task will be to stop it, to shut it off, so you can go to sleep after the gig."* This is the essence of pure improvisation. It is jumping into or onto a wave of the creative life force that then expresses itself through you, rather than your making anything happen.

Once you have been caught by a natural rhythm in Autokinetics, recognize that this is the opening to a flow of improvised expression. Allow the energy to express itself as it calls you to do so. You can make dancelike movements, body postures, and expressions or use your voice to make sounds, whether they be musical or not. You may chirp or whistle like a bird, growl like a lion, sing operatic nonsense, or sing scat to made-up melodies. Again, there is no right or wrong action. The important difference here is between unnatural and natural action. You know the latter because it is spontaneous and effortless, and it is not distracted from attending to the ongoing expression.

I used Autokinetics with a woman who is the director of a theater in North Carolina. Her career is partly devoted to the exploration of improvised sounds that can be made with the human voice and how they can bring forth life energy. In working with sound, it is important to know that a forced, unnatural sound will deflate your energy, whereas an effortless sound that seems to be voiced on its own without any exercise of will or intent on your part is very empowering. In fact, we found that when a body moving in sync with the life force is accompanied by improvised vocalizations, there is an amplification of our life energy.

The energizing aspects of making sound have been known for centuries. Tibet, China, India, Bali, and numerous other cultures have long used the production of musical tones to bring about life energy experiences. They developed various ways of producing sounds from

---

*Transcribed in the jazz newsletter, *Letter from Evans*, November–December 1991, p. 9.

many places along our body string, demonstrating that sound may come from the throat, the solar plexus, the base of the spine, or the crown of the head. Our body is both a vibrating string and an air column that is perfectly made to produce natural movements and sounds, which in turn bring us more readily into the flow of life's energy.

Here are some examples of natural body motions that sometimes take place when people take a ten-minute energy break and practice their Autokinetics. These movements are shown to you to give you some idea of the kind of movements that might emerge. Do not purposefully do them as you would calisthenics. They are not exercises for you to perform but simply examples of the range of movements that you might find yourself falling into and exploring.

The movement in Figure 2 is done rhythmically, with arms going outward and moving as if they were wings.

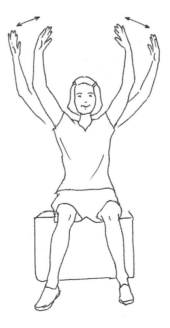

In Figure 3, your arms and hands move as if you were doing some form of martial arts.

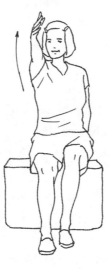

There are also variations of moving your feet as if you were doing a tap dance while sitting (Figure 4).

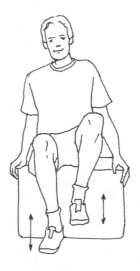

In the movement in Figure 5, you flutter all of your fingers as if they were being charged with an electrical current.

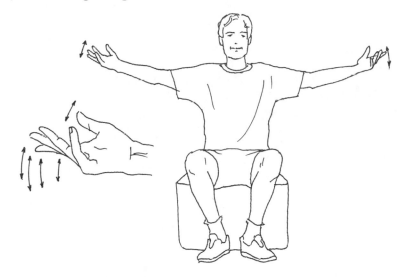

You can do the twist while you sit (Figure 6).

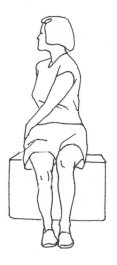

Various bouncing movements can be generated by placing one foot on a bench or chair (Figure 7).

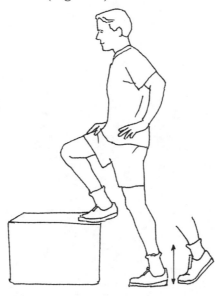

You may find yourself hitting the floor with your heels, alternating between the left and right feet (Figure 8). According to the tradition of *seiki-jutsu,* this helps rejuvenate your brain and contributes to bringing about a sense of balance.

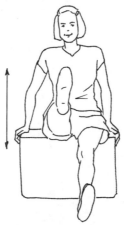

Beyond Right versus Wrong Movements   Oscar Peterson, the extraordinary jazz pianist, once commented that to the pure improvisationalist, there is no such thing as a "wrong note." There are only outcomes, each of which can be integrated into the flow of an ongoing sequence of notes. If a jazz master like Thelonious Monk hits an unexpected note, then he celebrates it as a surprise and uses it to take him in an unanticipated direction. Every note is accepted as perfect and as contributing to the ongoing creative flow. As any music lover can tell you, listening to someone play all the right notes without heart and soul is somehow wrong, whereas playing a supposedly wrong note with heart and soul is musically right.

The implication of this for you is that you must enter into the natural movements with no care for the distinction between right and wrong. If you make what you think are the right movements, but they don't feel effortless, then it is not natural. However, if you make some movements that you can't imagine being right, because they are so subtle, or ridiculous, or without meaning, but they feel effortless, then you are really right on. Don't fret over doing the right thing. Be natural, and all will flow as it should. Also, do not allow any self-admonishment of any kind. Instead, give in to being free to express yourself. Expression is a state of release, whether it be in sculpture, acting, writing, painting, dance, speaking, music, or simple movement.

When you do not feel a natural flow of movement, or if you lose the rhythm, don't worry about it. Wait it out, return to step one, and start again. Your Autokinetics practice will have its own rhythms, going in and out of the rhythmic flow, and this will happen more on some days than others. Respect and even cherish the moments when you are out of the flow, because those are the opportunities for you to experiment with new ways of bringing you back into it.

Tapping into Creativity Through step two, as your expression flows naturally, your whole being will move a step closer to being tuned to the life force. Here you will learn firsthand that the life force and the creative force are intertwined. Tapping into your creative energy is none other than hitting the vein of the life force. This explains why a complete immersion in a creative project is so rejuvenating.

Sometimes the creative source we tap into seems to be outside of our conscious knowledge base. For example, one of the fascinating outcomes that can occur when you practice Autokinetics on a regular basis is the spontaneous performance of a technical movement from an ancient tradition that you know little or nothing about. This may take place with absolute perfection even though you may not be aware of what you are doing. It can happen quite frequently, and it brings out an important point about the work. Most instruction in the ancient practices of energy work, such as tai chi and other martial arts, begins by teaching you very specific patterns of movement. This standardized choreography must be memorized by your mind and body and prac- ticed until it is perfectly realized. After many years of devoted practice, if you are lucky, a miraculous event takes place. You forget everything you have learned and fall into doing the patterns without any effort or conscious intent.

The same kind of educational process steers the way we teach people to play music. Years of study are spent learning the notes, the- ory, scales, and technique until various memorized scores are com- pletely mastered. You persevere with the hope that one day you will forget all the technique that was drilled into you and allow the music to play itself naturally and automatically.

Similarly, imagine being a baseball pitcher and constructing your- self a wire tunnel that goes from the pitching mound all the way to the strike zone at home plate. After building this tunnel, you practice throwing the ball down it so that it zooms across the plate. This is the way we usually learn—by building the tunnel, structure, or template that holds the action we wish to express and then throwing ourselves into it until we come out the other end with the desired result.

What this idea suggests is that our learning process is usually upside down. We build the template first and then try to force ourselves into it. After learning to do so, we hope that the process will just happen naturally. Unfortunately, most students give up before they get to any experience of spontaneously making music or throwing a perfect strike.

The alternative approach is to assume that the pattern for the activity we desire is already present as a field of energy and that we simply have to resonate with it. In doing so we move through it in an effortless way. Here we do not conceptualize ourselves as having anything to do with hard-earned achievement or making something happen; we think more in terms of cooperating and flowing with a natural pattern that holds the performance we desire.

I have met factory workers, mechanics, and repair personnel who intuitively do this. Whether operating a drill press, tightening a bolt, or replacing a wire, some of these workers have learned that their work is a powerful practice of learning to "feel yourself" around and through a machine. I believe that their natural knack for fixing things comes from their having learned to sense and work with the fields of energy of the machines they encounter. Their hands literally become guided to the trouble spot. If you listen to master mechanics talk about their work, it's not that different from listening to old-time dowsers explain how they find water in the ground. It's all about acquiring the "natural feel for the thing," or—as I'm discussing it—learning to enter into the energy field that relates all of the interconnected parts within it.

Once when I was teaching in Lubbock, Texas, I taught Autokinetics to an oil worker. Whenever he took an energy break, he saw himself as an oil pump that had to rock back and forth in order to bring up the energy of life. As a human pump, he orchestrated himself to fall into the rhythm and motions that would prime the natural flow of energy into his body. He enabled me to see this practice as a "pumping of energy" that takes place when we allow our body movements to be as rhythmic as an oil pump standing over a Texan's oil field.

As you learn to bring forth natural movements of your body, see them as drilling openings that bring forth the creative currents of improvisational expression. Here you literally perform yourself, bringing whatever you hold inside into an outward display of motion and sound.

To summarize: In step one, you move yourself to find a natural rhythm. There you feel the pulse that marks the true beginning of Autokinetics. Once this rhythmic pulse is established, your body is called to enter step two, the free-form expression of body movement and sound. This activity is an experience of releasing and transforming your inner feelings, thoughts, and intuitions into the outer expression of live performance. Some of my clients think of step two as an emptying process or a purging of all that is inside them through acting it out.

Step two accomplishes what meditation aims for when it requests that you empty yourself. Autokinetics does this by allowing your "inner world" to dance itself into the "outer world." This dancing and sounding yourself out may take anywhere from two to eight minutes, and it is the final preparation for moving you into the tuning zone, the place where you get charged with the life force.

Step Three: Enter the Tuning Zone

When you are captured by a natural movement and allow it to be voiced through improvisational expression, think of yourself as a surfer catching a wave. In surfing you wait for a wave to come along, you attempt to catch it and balance yourself on it, and you are carried forward on an invigorating ride. Similarly, the natural movement that you aim to bring forth in the first two steps of Autokinetics is analogous to waiting for a wave or current that you try to ride.

Where will this ride take you? Straight into step three, in which you enter a tuning zone that energizes you. Here you become less conscious of what you are doing and feel completely absorbed in a trancelike state. This is where you fall into a frequency that resonates with the pulse of earth's life force and find yourself being charged with vitality.

If you become too thrilled by what's happening and then start gloating over it, you will pull yourself out of the zone. Similarly, if you start analyzing what is going on or worrying about whether it will last or hoping that it will really help you, you will get beached. Your mind must stay focused on the experience at hand and not drift upward in a hot-air balloon of observation and reflection. Stay grounded in the experience, and do not permit your mind to float above it.

The groundedness I am speaking of is pure absorption in the experience at hand. In Autokinetics you are purposefully setting out to bring yourself into trancelike absorption, the tuning zone where you resonate with the pulse of life's energy. This tuning zone is what Zen Buddhism refers to as your "center of being," the place where your life becomes completely in tune with the energy of life.

When you fall into the natural rhythm of step one, you will feel as though you are starting to move toward a state of trance. When the motion grabs you in step two and moves you automatically, it stills your mind, relaxes your body, and brings you to a deeper level of consciousness. All this happens without any effort on your part. You enter step three when a trancelike state is accompanied by an inner vibration or pulse that beats at the same rate as that of the life force. This is the tuning zone. It is the same place that meditators, seekers of higher consciousness, and mystics are seeking in their practice and their journey. This is one of the most amazing outcomes of the practice. Without any effort, you enter realms that meditative techniques often take years to achieve.

Autokinetics teaches your mind to ride along with the natural flow of life. You want a mind that is a good horseback rider, a mind that knows how to feel the movements of life and is so attentive to them that you feel inseparable from life's motion. This is how you ride the spirit of life and allow it to take you into the altered state of consciousness that comes over you when you enter the tuning zone.

It doesn't take long to have a good ride with Autokinetics. Just a few minutes—sometimes five or ten, or longer if you want—will be enough to tune you in to natural living and fill you with a sense of being energized. Therefore, you need to give yourself only ten minutes here and there throughout the day to benefit from this technique. As you clear more space for this practice, it will become easier over time, and its effects will gradually become more immediate and powerful. Over the years you will find that the practice becomes an automatic part of your life, so that you start giving yourself an energy break whenever there is a need for you to be tuned and energized.

When you practice Autokinetics, you will notice that each time you do it, it naturally comes to a close. You come out of your trance and feel calm, blissful, and ready to start life all over again. As this reentry into everyday life begins to take place, allow your movements to gently slow down and come to a stop. When the movement ceases, apply your fingers to your eyeballs again and gently press on them as shown in Figure 1 on page 45. This time the eye pressure sends the message that your energy break is completed.

In Japan this exercise is believed not only to bring the life force into your body but also to push away the tiredness that has accumulated in it. I also believe that it is good to express a heartfelt "thank you" at the end of the practice, as an expression of your appreciation for its ancient roots.

Don't Forget Your Energy Break: The Daily Practice of Autokinetics

When you begin using Autokinetics, I suggest that you schedule it at least once a day. You may want an energy break when you first get up in the morning, or before you retire at night, or during a midday recess. Start in small steps, and don't overdo it. It is better for you to start with a one-minute effortless session than push yourself to have lengthy sessions of disciplined, hardworking effort. Remember that what you are doing is *effortless* motion. If it feels like a drag, then you are working too much.

As you fall more naturally into this effortless practice, allow it to increase at its own rate. You will eventually begin adding energy breaks throughout the day and night as you feel you need them. Some breaks may only last a minute or two, whereas others may last five, ten, or twenty minutes. As you learn to feel your body call for a tuning, you will find a way to do it, even if it means taking a brief time-out from work and finding a quiet place to do your movements, whether it be in a public park, in the privacy of a restroom, or at your work area. You will learn that there are subtle ways of performing it.

At the end of an energy break, you will often feel invigorated and more able to meet the subsequent challenges that await you. This sense is not of manic, wild energy, but of energy that is calm and confident. It is an inner energy that fills you with the sense that your life has a special purpose. One of my clients in Louisiana uses Autokinetics with her baby son when he wakes up in the middle of the night. She sits with him in her rocking chair and gently rocks herself into the tuning zone. To her amazement, she has found that her baby is more likely to go back to sleep when she focuses less on relaxing him and more on energizing herself. As she enters the tuning zone, her baby often goes back to sleep. Since Autokinetics brings you *calm* energy, it makes sense that it can help you or your baby fall asleep.

Another client, a computer programmer from Boulder, Colorado, said that he feels Autokinetics gives him a greater belief in himself, and that he practices it for the immediate confidence it gives him. Other clients are pleasantly surprised to discover that Autokinetics leaves them feeling less entangled in the daily issues and problems that surround them. It gives them a feeling of freedom and independence. Having done these movements for many years, I find that I feel a tingly sensation after a session, as if I had just been plugged into an electrical circuit. Other people who have used this technique for several years report the same kind of experience.

As you become familiar with this way of moving your body so that you are, in turn, moved by life, it will become as vital to your well-being as your sleep and diet. You will also appreciate the variety of ways you can integrate Autokinetics into your daily affairs. You do not always have to go through all the steps as I have defined them. The steps may eventually become one single step in which getting a rhythm, moving improvisationally, and going into the tuning zone all happen at the same time. You may find that in the middle of a business meeting you can initiate a tiny movement that is not perceptible to anyone, and then proceed to tune yourself to be more effective in the ongoing interactions and negotiations. This is already being done by business executives in Japan who have been taught *seiki-jutsu* and other energy techniques. Indeed, energy practices have become so widespread that they inspired a feature story in the business section of a recent issue of *The New York Times.*

Take some time to experiment with making the tiniest movements you can with Autokinetics. Discover how the size of the movement has little to do with the magnitude of the energizing effect, and how the smaller movements feel more like vibrations or a buzzing and tingling. Sometimes it may seem that these vibrations are taking place inside of you. As you learn to do Autokinetics with small movements which aren't perceived by others and which may even take place inside your body, the door will open for you to bring the energy break anywhere that you go during the course of your daily life.

One client, a successful salesman from Chicago, told me that he used Autokinetics as part of a strategy for making a sale in his business. Before he gave his final sales pitch, he would create a steady rhythmic movement of his right hand and allow himself to gently enter what he called the "sale zone." While in this state of calm energy, he would make his sales pitch. Without anyone knowing what he was doing, he made business deals while he was in an energized state of trance! He said that when he was through with his talk, he felt completely alive and invigorated. In his way, he took the most challenging aspect of his daily work and turned it into one of the most rewarding times of his life.

Autokinetics provides you with more than a once-a-day energy break that you add to your life. It is a way of breathing energy, vitality, and inspiration that can be used at any moment. Although you will learn how to work with this energy when you regularly sit down and do it, know that this will eventually lead to a time when you can do it under any circumstances and in any situation. You will find that whenever you need a boost from life, all you have to do is bring forth a little motion or vibration into your body and allow it to carry you into the tuning zone.

This gives you an edge in performing all the activities of your life—in both work and play. As you learn to energize yourself throughout the day with the natural movements your body desires to make, your physical well-being will be maximized, enabling you to have the healthy glow that characterizes all people who keep the life force flowing through their body. Your attitude and outlook will change, and you will become more filled with optimism and the belief that you can do the things you really want to accomplish. There is no better health supplement or technique of success than experiencing contact with the energy of life.

Time and time again I have seen people start using Autokinetics simply because they wanted more energy to get them through the day. They were undergoing their own personal energy crisis, and they didn't allow themselves even to fantasize or dream about a better life. They just wanted enough energy to survive. To their great delight, Autokinetics did more than return energy to their daily life. It took away the dark cloud that had kept them from seeing anything hopeful, and it showed them a new world of personal possibilities.

We have heard a lot about the benefits of positive thinking, and I join with all those who urge us to bring a more positive and resourceful perspective into our daily participation in life. I extend this advice to being more broadly understood as the pursuit of *positive energy resonances* that revitalize each of us in the course of our daily living. Finding and experiencing these resonances of positive energy throughout the day is part of what it means to live a charged life.

When you start using Autokinetics, I encourage you to go into each day with the desire to catch as many *energy tingles* as you can. A tingle is any vibratory body sensation that is naturally stimulated by a moment of inspiration. These may be brought about in an endless number of ways. Be on the lookout for someone's special smile, the glowing joy expressed between an older couple in love, an ecstatic strain of music that goes straight to your heart, or the unpredictable, delightful facial expressions of a child. Look differently at your natural surroundings and see if you can find the wind blowing a leaf in a way that is more masterly than any movement on the dance floor. Study the life of dogs and wonder why many mystics consider them enlightened beings. Open your hand to catch a raindrop or a snowflake and think about how your life would change if you did this on a regular basis. Become more mindful of where the best scents and tastes are hidden in your city. Go to a bakery and try using your nose in a more devoted way. Order one thing in a restauraunt and give great attention to its taste. Do these things as a means of helping yourself be tickled, touched, and tingled by the vital bounty of life. Appreciate the fact that this tingle is the current of the universal life force and that there are many simple ways to plug yourself into it by opening your sensory processes. Allow your ears, eyes, mouth, nose, hands, and body to find new ways of getting into contact with the life force.

I worked with a young actress from Los Angeles who loved to sing the well-known commercial jingle, "Give yourself a break today" and then add, "in vibrations." She felt that the whole technique really boiled down to being a way of bringing vibrations or pulsing movements into her body and that this tuned her to the life force. Whenever she felt the need for some energy or revitalization, she would instantly sing that line to herself and take a moment to initiate a movement or vibration that tuned her to life energy.

*   *   *   *   *   *   *   *   *

Autokinetics can now be summarized in a very simple way. Recall that earlier we discussed the body as analogous to a piano or guitar string, terming it a "body string." With this notion, energizing yourself is all about tuning your body string. This string, which roughly corresponds to the length of your spinal column, must be moved in order to be tuned. When it vibrates in sync with the frequency of the life force, you become energized. The technique for tuning yourself constitutes the three steps we have already reviewed, which can be expressed as follows in terms of being understood as the tuning of your body string:

1. Wiggle, shake, move, or vibrate your body string and allow that movement to have a natural rhythm.
2. Encourage your body string to freely dance and sing to its beat.
3. As the dance falls deeply into the beat, you enter the hypnotic-like tuning zone. There your body string resonates with the energy of life and brings you fresh vitality.

Children naturally dance their body string to the energizing beat of life, but adults too often allow their string to be pulled out of tune by the stresses of everyday life and then find themselves truly bent out of shape. Get back to the energizing beat of life and allow it to move you in the right direction. I don't care how much therapy, medicine, or self-help you get—if your string isn't tuned, nothing may help. In fact, adding more movement to an already out-of-tune string may bring forth only more disturbing noise. Before you do anything to yourself or allow anyone else to do something to you, first take an energy break and get yourself tuned. Get tuned and see how easily everything else starts to fall into place when you have the energy of life moving through you.

As you become more familiar with falling into the movements of the universal life force, you will find your own unique modifications and methods that maximize its effectiveness for you. What is freeing about this technique is its insistence that you never worry over whether you are doing it right. Every way is right as long as you use it to bring you into the natural, effortless motions of the life force. In this regard, you begin at the final lesson—learning to be natural. You do not have to wait years or even decades learning what you will eventually have to throw away. You begin where you want to end and then, with each passing week and year, you move more into the natural way of living.

There was a remarkable teacher in Boston named Madame Chalaff who taught many famous pianists, such as Keith Jarrett and Herbie Hancock. She began with one simple lesson: how to play one note perfectly and effortlessly. Once you got that lesson, you had most of what she felt was important about making music—or, I should say, about how music can effortlessly make itself through you. In the beginning lessons she encouraged her students not to practice longer than five or ten minutes. Any more time would encourage them to drift away from effortless playing. The same lesson holds for you. In the beginning you should never perform the technique too long, because this would take you into a frame of mind that is too purposeful, serious, effortful, and unnatural. Always perform your Autokinetics with the underlying commitment to having it become as natural as play. Practice the energizing of your life with the intention of becoming more interwoven with the vitality of nature.

I encourage you to take an occasional energy break in the same state of mind as that of an indigenous person who enters a ceremony.

Here the technique and the art of moving naturally, the body's motion and the mind's flow, the soulful expression of yourself and the presence of the creative spirit, all flow together with no separation. In this web of life, you will find endless energy, inspiration, and dreams that carry you into the life that you most deeply desire.

CHAPTER THREE

Entering the Charged Life

■――――――――――――――――

Optimizing the quality of your life, from the viewpoint of life energy, is all about keeping yourself tuned to those resonances that keep the life force flowing through you. This idea brings forth a radical shift in how we think of taking care of ourselves.

With the practice of Autokinetics you can go into each day with the understanding that every single experience that comes your way is an energy opportunity that you can use to enhance your well-being. I'm referring to both everyday routines and surprises. Literally everything that happens to you, whether you see it as good or bad, is an opportunity for you to evolve your participation with the life force. The challenge for you is to learn how to relate to all the events of your life, both the disappointments and the personal victories, in a way that keeps you tuned and moving with life's energizing currents.

When you practice the energy way, you will find that there are some basic insights that help keep you in the tuning zone, the place where vitality naturally springs forth:

- Although you don't have to hold on to the way in which energy is delivered to you, never resist the energy of life that comes your way. For instance, if you are angry with someone, take the energy from the interaction, but release the anger. Or if you find yourself love-struck with a character in a movie, take the energy, but release the fantasy.

- When you feel stirred up, whether in a good or a bad way, allow your body to move. Never sit still when the force of life rocks your boat. Move your body with the currents of its energy and allow this impact to dance you into the tuning zone.
- The energy of life is simply energy. It has no connotations of good or bad and is free of judgment. The more you see life as energy, instead of a series of good and bad situations, the easier it will be for you to accept your experience as an energy event.

When we move away from living life as energy, we tend to sit down and get into an internal immobilizing state of overevaluating and over-judging our past, present, and future. The result is a drain of energy and a sinking feeling of bitterness and hopelessness.

Carrying out Autokinetics on a daily basis is probably the healthiest thing you can do for your life. In Japan I met dozens of people in all walks of life, from scientists and engineers to artists, business executives, and retired people, who practiced their movement exercises daily. Most of them ate whatever they wanted, had no regimented exercise program, and lived their life free from overregulation and restrictions. With simply the natural movements that took place when they sat down on their *seiki* bench, they were able to fill their lives with vitality and energy and bring forth the healthy and youthful glow that characterizes the natural state of general well-being.

Once you become familiar on a daily basis with the natural motions that open you to the energizing currents of the life force, as demonstrated in Chapter Two, you will find that you have a powerful resource for transforming your everyday life. There are numerous ways to bring the self-revitalizing technique of Autokinetics into the activities and challenges of each day. You can do variations of Auto-kinetics at the workplace, within family life, or during sports and recreation. In this chapter, I will show you how living a charged life can bring new resources, understanding, and discoveries to every area of your life.

Protecting Yourself from the Energy Drain

Everyone is familiar with the experience of having energy dissipate or feeling life's vitality being drained away. Sometimes we encounter people who seem to zap our energy. While it may be true that our interactions with them are draining, this doesn't necessarily mean that they are to blame. It is the pattern of interaction, the relationship, or—in our language—the *resonance* between you that leads to an energy issue. What you want to avoid is a "draining resonance."

Here's an example. I once met a recently divorced counselor from Miami who seemed to drain the energy out of everyone she ever talked to. I felt it happen when I was with her. What I noticed about her interaction was that she always talked, and she talked nonstop. It was impossible to get a word in, and if you did manage to squeeze in a sentence, she would immediately cut you off. She didn't hesitate to give you advice, but she never allowed anyone else to have any air time. In addition, there was seldom a moment of lightness or humor in her presence, and little activity. It was all talk, including talk about action, but little opportunities for real physical movement and tactile contact. When all these ingredients are thrown together—a rigid monologue, absence of humor, and little physical movement—I have found that the situation is ripe for a real energy drain.

All you can do in such a situation is try to ask for some air time that breaks up the monologue and then try moving toward a dialogue. The other thing you can try is to introduce some humor or absurdity.

Tell a joke or simply start laughing and tell the other person about the last time something made you laugh. And finally, get up and move about. Move your body so it isn't caught in the deadly position of being a static listening device. And if none of these things work, then get out of the situation as quickly and as gracefully as you can. Beware of the energy drain. It is a real experience, and it can lead to a headache, body aches, and colossal fatigue.

Recall that whenever two waves interfere with each other, it is possible for them to cancel each other out. This creation of interference is illustrated when you drop three pebbles into a shallow round pan of water. When you do this, you see that each stone hits the water and sends waves spreading across the pan. When the waves cross each other, they create complex patterns of interference. If you think of each wave as having a high and low point—or a mountaintop and a valley—you can see that when the high point of one wave interacts with the low point of another wave, they create a flat spot: that is, they cancel each other. When one person does all the talking and completely dominates an interaction, while the other person remains still and silent, one or both people may feel drained. Their nonshifting and opposite ways of being present cancel each other out.

When you feel drained in the presence of another person, it is partly due to the fact that the two of you are canceling out each other's waves of life force. To increase the height and depth of each wave requires that the two waves match and line up together. Again, when this happens, the combination results in increasing the amplitude or energy of each wave. One way to do this involves finding out how to meet someone on your particular frequency. When you do this, you may be surprised to find yourself recharged by the interaction. You must tune yourself in to the other person's frequency as if you were searching for a radio station. You have to turn your inner dial to find the frequency at which there is some music available for your listening pleasure. Fortunately, most human beings are not limited to one frequency. Like any decent radio set, people carry several stations, and there usually is one that plays the kind of music that speaks to you. Ideally, *each* of you will try to tune in to the other and find some mutually satisfying station. I will acknowledge, however, that sometimes you will be unable to find any music that you are comfortable hearing. In such a case you may have to excuse yourself from the situation and look for another person to tune in with—as was the case with the monotonous counselor.

I once worked with a couple who believed that they loved each other but found their time together to be completely exhausting. They had different careers and separate social lives and couldn't find anything to talk about that was mutually interesting. Since they seemed to have no common interest, I suggested that they find out what they both agreed was uninteresting. With little effort they were able to admit that neither one of them was very interested in cooking. I then told them to spend at least ten minutes a day discussing why they weren't interested in cooking. This shared uninterest in cooking helped bring them into a positive resonance with one another. To their great surprise, they enjoyed talking about why neither of them liked to cook. Learning to be on the same frequency in what they disliked helped them learn to be on the same frequency in other parts of their marriage.

Creating Resonance   Seeing our interaction with others as the *creation of a resonance* suggests that we have more flexibility in how we communicate. Rather than stay in any fixed role, we need to explore the ways in which we can change our presence so as to help bring forth the kind of resonance that benefits each of us. Again, this stops us from lazily judging and dismissing people and moves us toward being explorers and inventors of many different ways to relate to another person.

There are some people with whom we will benefit more from being still and quiet, but with other people an optimal interaction may involve more of an exchange of words and sounds and movements. These patterns of interaction may also change within a particular relationship: part of the time the two of you will need to be more silent, whereas at other times you will require more activity to bring out a vitalizing resonance.

Not only does this understanding apply to your interaction with other people; it also holds for how you relate to your work, leisure, everyday routines, and activities. Every aspect of your life can now be assessed in terms of how you resonate with it. Instead of asking whether you have the right job, you should explore the resonances that you create in your work space. This shift in perspective gives you more options for energizing your life.

Similarly, your home life can be examined with respect to how you bring forth various patterns of resonance. It is important that you begin cultivating the idea of yourself as a creator of waves of energy, waves that interact with other waves and bring forth resonances, some of which are energizing while others are draining.

Joining the Other Person's Reality   The key to avoiding the energy drain is to make sure that you don't stay stuck in a resonance that cancels out or drains away your life force. To help protect yourself from these life-draining experiences, keep this simple advice in mind: Always join the reality of the other person. This does not mean that you have to accept or practice what others believe. It is an invitation for you to enter into their worldview, their way of seeing, hearing, feeling, and intuiting. This includes using the metaphors, understanding, and language that they bring to your encounter. If you meet people who talk business, then join them in that worldview. Don't talk to them in a psychological way or with spiritually loaded words. To do so would be to risk canceling each other out and would result in your going home drained of energy.

Accomplished therapists are very familiar with this technique of accepting and utilizing the language of the other person. They will speak the metaphors of their client rather than persuade the client to speak in any specialized therapeutic lingo. This attitude of "joining with the other" is always a great way to stimulate a good energy connection and a powerful way to prevent the interaction from draining you. You may be tempted to think that this is giving in to other people, and that this surrender places you in a one-down position to them so that they are more able to exploit and drain you. It may seem paradoxical that this is not the case. When you step into other people's worlds, you meet them on their ground and they are immediately put at ease and comforted by your natural presence in their experiential home. This frees them to be more natural and often moves them to be more open and accepting of you. When you accept and enter into another's way of communicating, there is an immediate sense of joining that is felt by each of you, and this buzz of connection facilitates your moving toward giving energy to one another.

I helped a thirty-year-old accountant from New Jersey who had an impossible boss. No matter what he did, his boss was always critical, overly serious, and never available to listen to another person's side of the story. Work had become a major energy drain, and the employee was beginning to consider leaving the company. I asked him to try one final thing before he quit, to do some sleuthing in order to find out what his boss liked to do when he wasn't at work. I suggested that he might examine the photos and pictures on his office walls to see if they provided any clues and to also drop some innocent questions that might tempt his boss to open up and share his passionate interests.

After some brief detective work, the employee called me and said that his boss had pictures of horses throughout his office. When the man asked his boss about whether he followed the horse races, his boss had responded with the most positive reaction he had ever seen him offer. As it turns out, his boss was totally into horse racing and was frustrated with his life because he wanted more than anything else to have a farm and raise prize racehorses. From that moment on, his boss waited each day to be asked something about horses. The two of them began following the races in the sports pages, and the employee became filled with new energy and vitality, simply because he had found a frequency where he could positively resonate with his boss.

When you approach what you perceive as the mundane activities of daily living, whether in your home or at your workplace, you should also meet them on their own terms. For example, accept the routine of washing your laundry as an act of importance. Respect it with the Zenlike attitude that it holds the possibility of a moment of teaching, life enhancement, and revitalization. Perhaps it affords you the gift of a few quiet moments in a highly scheduled day. The important thing is not to complain about its being a boring, trivial aspect of your life. This too easily leads to doing the task as a chore that drains you of energy. Step into it as an opportunity to create an energizing resonance. In this practice you will find that all of your life, including its dirty laundry, becomes an opportunity for revitalizing yourself.

It's Natural to Fall Out of Tune   Even if you have the right attitude about life's energy, you will still have to be on the lookout for the kind of events that can all too easily take you out of tune. When these events show up, try to break away from your old habits of getting emotionally caught up in them or endlessly worrying and obsessing over how to understand the situation or solve the problem. Instead, curb your reactive emoting, worrying, and calculating and immediately set about to get yourself retuned. Here are some of the normal things that typically happen to everyone and tend to immediately throw us out of tune:

- *Bad news.* Someone tells us about an unexpected outcome that we had not imagined would take place, such as illness, a difficult relationship, or loss of job.
- *A little accident.* It's not only the big ones that throw us out of whack. Minor fender benders and falls on the sidewalk can throw you out of tune.
- *Deprivation.* Not getting what you really need can tilt your system. This applies not only to nutrition, rest, exercise, and money, but to healthy conversation, sex, quiet time, and dance time.
- *Too much of a good thing.* Sometimes we don't know when to push the plate aside, when to leave the party, when to stop celebrating, or when to turn off the television set. Overindulgence in any aspect of daily life can detune our system as easily as deprivation.
- *The blues.* Too much time spent on personal evaluation almost always inspires your inner judge to condemn your life as a wasted effort.
- *Not enough laughter.* Don't deprive yourself of healing laughter, one of the best natural processes of tuning yourself. Too much seriousness is a drain on the life force.

- *Success.* Success as well as defeat can catch you off guard and pull you out of tune.

Keep your eyes open for any of these episodes that could show up in your life. If they do, call a time-out and step aside from what you are doing in order to have an energy break and get yourself retuned. Do not fight or resist the unanticipated event that has manifested itself, but find a way to utilize it so that its energy is redirected toward helping you find an energizing resonance.

For instance, if you find out that you have just lost some money, you can take notice of how you begin to get upset and, as you do so, throw a conceptual curveball into this emotional process. Say something to yourself that doesn't deny or fight against what has happened. Do not say anything like, "Things will get better" or "I'm sure I'll get over it." Instead *join with* whatever has smacked you in the face—in this case, the idea, "I am losing my money"—and then *exaggerate it* into some absurd statements such as, "This is the beginning of the end. When all my money is gone, I'll be able to go on that walkabout in Australia." Perhaps your sense of the absurd may carry you in another direction: "I wonder if I should give away the rest of my money so that I won't fear losing it." In these responses you use mental judo to flow with the force that came upon you, and to continue moving that force toward some fantasized or absurd end. This helps free you from being stuck in worry over the situation and gives you new energy to address the problems.

One of the things that happens when we are shocked by really bad news is that we start to feel an overwhelming sense of panic, a sense that our life is out of control. When you are suddenly fired from your job, lose a relationship, or are threatened with a lawsuit, there is usually an avalanche of fear and worry that starts rolling over you. This panic may erupt into a full-blown anxiety attack, where your body actually feels feverish, moving back and forth between chills and sweating. You may also feel as if you are dizzy and may even believe that you are having a heart attack. All of these panicky reactions tempt us to take our problems inside our mind, where we enter a cyclone of whirling thoughts and emotions. In this fear-driven state, the more we think and worry about the situation, the worse we feel and the more drained we are of the life force.

There is a way out that requires us to take the energy from a panic response—the same energy that makes us feel dizzy—and externalize it so that our body is permitted to move in a natural way. Don't take the energy inside, where it will whirl you into the energy drain. Instead, take an energy break and use the three-step technique of Autokinetics—let the energy move your body so that the panic is released while your whole being is brought back into the tuning zone, the place that is always ready to help you in times of great need. When your body is moved by the energy that is stirred up by bad news, it will dance the energy out, free your mind from an overload of worry, and help bring about a state of peace and calm.

The advice I give to you for protecting yourself from being drained of energy runs counter to most recommendations given by others for psychological or spiritual protection. Typically, you are told to set up a wall of protection—either a conceptual boundary or an internally visualized brick fortress—and are then told to believe that this will help keep the outside harmful stuff from entering you. I believe that any attitude of resistance sets you up to create a resonance that is draining. This is not about stopping the flow of bad energy into us or holding in the flow of good energy. It is about the quality of resonance we have with one another. Interactions that are inspired by resistance invite disharmonious resonances that are more likely to drain us. The perennial advice to love our enemies moves us to create a resonance with others that enables all parties to benefit from the vital life force pulsing through the interaction.

In summary, the best protection against being drained of energy is to stop fighting life itself. Join life by exploring the endless ways of bringing forth a vitalizing resonance. Step into the shoes of others. Speak their language. Adopt the attitude that you must find the rhythm or pulse of life in every situation that you encounter so that you can resonate with it in a positive way.

The hunt for an inspired resonance is the playful spirit of a good jazz ensemble. Whenever one instrumentalist offers a melodic line, another musician is free to join it and play with it as well. The musicians feed off of each other's energy and find themselves deeply revitalized by the experience. Similarly, you must see the whole of life as a kind of never-ending jazz performance that keeps throwing you a musical line to play with. If you enter into the spirit of improvisational play, you will find the resonances that invigorate and inspire the performance of your life, and of the life of those who are playing with you.

Activating the Inborn Ability to Heal Yourself

Every time you perform Autokinetics, you bring healing energy into your body. That is, you bring forth a natural condition of health and well-being. In addition to this general process of daily healing, there are more specific acts of healing that have to do with trying to cure the aches, pains, and illnesses that sometimes come to us. The therapeutic, healing benefits of moving the life force through your body have been heralded by some contemporary western practitioners. In his superb book *Spontaneous Healing*, Dr. Andrew Weil tells the story of his search for great healers, a journey that took him around the world but led him back to his own backyard—where he discovered his mentor, the osteopath Dr. Robert Fulford.

What makes Dr. Fulford unique in Western medicine is that he is the perfect embodiment of the old-time family doctor with a warm and caring demeanor. But what may surprise you is that he rarely prescribes medicine. His practice, described in his book *Dr. Fulford's Touch of Life: The Healing Power of the Natural Life Force,* relies almost entirely upon finding a way to move the life force through your body, particularly in the places where it is partially or completely blocked. Dr. Fulford believes that bringing the universal life force into our bodies is the best medicine for helping us get through the challenges and stresses of our time. He is referring both to the use of this energy as a way of maintaining a general state of well-being and to its use as a therapeutic approach to helping cure disease and illness.

The traumas of our life, whether they be from viral infections, physical blows, or emotional shocks, throw us out of tune and may lead us into mental suffering and physical disease. We too often limit ourselves to adopting a defensive attitude and set out to eradicate the surface symptoms. The surest road to recovery and health, however, is through tuning your whole being.

The most evolved view of healing recognizes that symptoms are usually signals of a deeper systemic pattern that may not be perceptible or recognized by either medical, psychological, or psychic diagnosis. Any overfocus on symptoms and disease isolates you from the whole field of life energy that is the web of your healing. If you move into a naturally tuned state, this field will activate all the inner healing processes of your body and turn on the natural healing power that arises from the energy of life. This is the highest level of healing.

I am not suggesting that people stop using the offerings of modern medicine and instead rely exclusively upon an energy technique. What I am saying is that all healing, all therapies, and all medicines are optimally effective whenever they are able to facilitate the flow of the life force. Dr. Elmer Green, director emeritus at the Voluntary Controls Program at the Menninger Clinic in Topeka, Kansas, proposes that alternative or complementary medicine—and, I would emphasize, energy healing—can adequately treat about 70 percent of all the complaints that are brought to medical doctors. I think that treatments for the remaining 30 percent, which may (or may not) require the more dramatic interventions of surgery and prescribed medication, will be greatly enhanced by treatment within a context that understands and promotes the healing power of the life force.

Today a cooperative spirit is beginning to develop between medical doctors and energy practitioners. At Columbia University Hospital, the energy healer Julie Mott lays her hands on the patient in the operating room as a heart transplant is going on. In the area of medical research, Dr. Robert Becker, professor of orthopedics at the Upstate Medical Center in Syracuse, New York, found that the introduction of energy that pulses at around eight cycles per second will help bone fractures and injuries heal more rapidly. More research and more therapeutic exploration await us in these directions. With the formation of the Office of Alternative Medicine at the National Institute of Health, there are strong signs that the medical community will continue its reawakening to the most traditional form of medicine and healing, which has been around for thousands of years.

When people struggling with a disease ask me for help, I never challenge the treatment given to them by their doctors and alternative practitioners. I simply say that there is nothing better than getting some life force into their bodies, doing so with the simple and gentle movements of Autokinetics. For instance, an older woman with breast cancer came to me at a conference in Santa Clara, California, and asked to learn Autokinetics. I explained that its practice might help her medical treatments do their job, because when her body is filled with energy, the healing power of life itself is able to amplify and maximize the beneficial effects of all therapeutic interventions. Medicine and surgery, I went on to say, work best on a body that is receiving a daily dose of life energy. This helps the body respond positively to the corrective adjustments and procedures of both conventional and non-conventional medical practices. The woman started taking energy breaks, faithfully doing her Autokinetics, and subsequently developed a more positive attitude and response to the treatment that her doctors were giving her. Fortunately for her, she was able to find the healing she had hoped for and returned to her daily life with a strong sense of recovery and health.

Experiencing Healing

Hand Dowsing   One of the amazing things that happens to people when they take an energy break and practice Autokinetics is that the body begins to learn how to heal itself, to become its own therapist. This often begins with your hands feeling pulled to move over various parts of your body. When that happens, feel free to pat, gently slap, massage, vibrate, poke, shake, move, and touch yourself in any way you feel drawn to explore. Allow your hands to *dowse* your body. As you learn to give them their own mind, they will fall into natural movements that help activate more healing experiences for you.

I worked with a woman who taught nursing in Toronto, and she immediately began seeing the therapeutic benefits of Autokinetics. After a year of doing it, she found that her daily practice became like a self-massage session. Her hands would work on her own body and bring relief to the aches and pains that were brought about by her workday. As she taught the practice to others, they, too, began reaping its therapeutic benefits. They found that the more that they did the technique, the more finely tuned they became to sensing where their hands should go and how they should touch their own bodies. Autokinetics itself became the vehicle for teaching them what to do. This learning happened automatically, without any textbook.

When you do Autokinetics for the purpose of self-healing, do not get caught in the trap of responding only to your obvious aches and pains. For example, if you have a sore calf muscle, then don't limit yourself to just reaching over and massaging it in an overly purposeful way. Sometimes our pains are best treated by therapeutically touching another part of the body. I'll never forget the time I worked with Troup Matthews, a practitioner of the Alexander Method, a classic approach to body movement. I complained of a neck pain, and he started moving my ankles. To my great surprise the neck pain went away. When we have a localized pain, we too easily forget that our body is a whole system. As many of the Asian traditions remind us, we are one organ made up of interrelated parts. With this in mind, step aside from any thinking process that directs you only to the sore spots and allow your hands and body to move as they are naturally called to do so.

Echoes of Past Injury   Some of the following experiences may take place as healing occurs: You may have numbness in some parts of your body. You may even lose sensation in your hands, your head, or other body locations for a moment and then find that they start to tingle. This takes place because the life force is opening the pores of your skin and increasing the blood circulation at various places under your skin. It is a sign that the life force is moving through you. You may also experience some body aches, particularly in areas that correspond to old injuries. If you have historically struggled with stomachaches, headaches, arthritis, or other problems, they may be momentarily amplified as the life force intensifies the circulation of energy through those problematic areas.

Therapeutic Sweat   Also, if you practice the technique for at least ten to twenty minutes, you may find that the energy warms up your body. Some people sweat profusely after doing Autokinetics and find that this contributes to making them feel even more invigorated. In some ancient traditions, the sweat that flows from an energized body is regarded as a medicine and is wiped onto areas of the body that need healing. Accept the water of perspiration as a healthy sign that the life force is lighting a healing fire within you.

Finger Dancing   When you do Autokinetics, you may want to think of your fingers in the way that one of my clients suggests. She sees her fingers as miniature dancers that want to improvise some movement on the surface of her skin. With this image in mind, allow your body to dance with itself in a never-ending choreography of improvised motion. Similarly, the palms of your hands, your elbows, and feet can be used to move about on various body parts. Empty yourself of any preconception of how you should touch yourself, whether it be from ideas regarding massage, body work, or healing, and allow yourself to tinker, experiment, explore, and dowse as a way of bringing healing energy into yourself.

Shaking   Another healing movement you may want to explore is shaking. Experiment with wiggling your arms and hands and allowing this wiggling to become a vigorous shaking. Your body can shake from side to side, from front to back, or up and down. Think of how you have seen a dog shake after it got out of a lake or swimming pool. Try the same for your whole body. Discover whether shaking opens some natural, healing rhythms for you. (In Chapter Five of this book, I discuss how a variety of global healing traditions use shaking to move the life force through the body.)

When I was on my way to Africa to visit the Kalahari Bushmen, I was seated on the airplane next to a South African physician. He began talking about his career and said that he had been the doctor assigned to the movie *The Gods Must Be Crazy*, a comedy about the Bushmen. At one point during the shooting of the film, the star of the film was brought to him, in a condition no one understood. His body had gone into a deep shaking. He was in a deep trance and could not engage in conversation. Some quick tests were given, but no evidence could be found to explain his movements. What the doctor and medical staff did not know was that the Bushman had entered a healing state and was restoring his health and vitality. The next day the Bushman stopped shaking and was found to be completely revitalized and ready for work.

You don't have to shake as intensely as that Bushman, but it may be worthwhile for you to spend some time exploring the shaking body movements that might offer you new possibilities for self-healing. When you vibrate, shake, or rock, explore whether you are able to produce some natural sounds. Throughout the world, cultures that practice energy healing often find that the spontaneous voicing of sound is therapeutic. Allow your voice to sound its vibrations if this feels natural to you.

Vibrations of Beauty Another important consideration concerns where you choose to take your energy break. You should find a place that is uplifting and beautiful. Develop an attitude like that of the Navajo, who fill their lives with natural beauty and are fully aware that the "beauty way" is a sure path to spiritual healing and attunement. You, too, should value beauty in your life, whether it be in the way you dress, the words you speak, the presentation of your meals, the presence of art, or simply bringing home some flowers from time to time. Beauty lifts the vibrations of your life and facilitates the flow of healing energy in your home. It is a medicine that brings delight to all of your senses.

Find Your Own Way   Ultimately, the best advice anyone could give you is to find your own way and discover your own voice and your own healing touch. It doesn't matter whether your hands get cold or hot when you sit down to heal yourself. It doesn't matter whether you shake or are less active. Your vibrations may be realized on the inside rather than the outside. You may holler or be silent. Many roads, one for each of us, take us to the truth of how we can heal ourselves.

However, you may want to keep these guidelines in mind—all stemming from the basic tenets of Autokinetics—whenever you find yourself facing aches and pains or an illness and want to draw upon using the energy of life to facilitate your therapy and recovery:

- Allow the natural movements of Autokinetics to bring forth a spontaneous way of touching and moving yourself.
- Allow the self-healing movements to follow their own course, knowing that they may include massage-like expression, finger dancing, body shaking, vocalizations of sound, and other improvised therapeutic movements.
- Keep your mind still and allow your hands and body to have a mind of their own. Know that with practice your hands will

become dowsing instruments that will go wherever they need to go without any conscious direction.

- Practice your self-healing in a place of beauty that inspires you.
- Remind yourself of what is most essential about Autokinetics—that it is all about taking you into the tuning zone, the place where you resonate positively with the energy of life. When you are tuned with the life force, you activate your inner healing processes and draw upon the healing energy of life itself.

As you learn to heal your whole being—your body, mind, and soul—you will realize that you carry all of the healing powers you need within yourself, and that the truest practice is to awaken your own inner processes of healing. As Albert Schweitzer once put it: "Each person carries his own doctor inside him. . . . We are at our best when we give the doctor who resides within each patient a chance to go to work." Find the resonances that activate and awaken the healing energies that reside within you. Dedicate yourself to the unbending desire to tune your whole being. When your instrument is tuned, the healing vibrations may be voiced.

As I travel around the world teaching people how to use Autokinetics, it is always a tremendous pleasure to hear how many people in the audience find that their headaches and body aches sometimes disappear with their first experience of making natural movements. At Interface, a teaching center in Cambridge, Massachusetts, a teacher of philosophy was surprised and delighted that his chronic backache disappeared after one weekend of working with Autokinetics. His pain had been with him for over twenty years, and it had not responded to any kind of treatment. Yet a few attempts at moving with the life force were enough to move his pain away and show him the kind of miraculous outcomes that are possible when you move naturally with life.

I was once asked to work with a frail man suffering from liver disease. He was in the last weeks of his life and was so weak that he had to be carried on a stretcher. He had been a professional actor and had once played the lead role in the Broadway musical *Jesus Christ Superstar*. He was taken to New Paltz, New York, where Stephen and Robin Larson, the authors of Joseph Campbell's biography, helped me conduct a special healing ceremony for this dying man. We moved the pulse of life through his body and witnessed him regain his desire for life. He sang a song, cried out with joy, and voiced a fantasy about making love. The simple movements of life had showered him with pure delight, giving him a night free of pain and filled with ecstasy.

The vibrations of healing energy feel like the purest form of delight we can experience. Whether healing someone else or practicing the art of self-healing, know that this is an act of pleasure. It makes you tingle and vibrate with happiness about being alive. In this act, you carry no ill will or negative emotions but open yourself to the energy that lovingly heals without judgment or purpose. This feeling of bliss marks the presence of the perfectly tuned human being. It is our greatest gift to one another and to ourselves.

A Moving Meditation

The purest forms of meditation also take you into the tuning zone and help revitalize your life. Most meditators learn that if you are told to be still and quiet your mind, a paradox often takes place. You find that your mind doesn't want to be still and that your body feels fidgety. Your mind will chase itself in circles, thinking about what it means not to think, or worrying about the fact that you can't stop worrying, or repetitively viewing replays of past events and future strategies.

Your mind and body simply don't want to be still. The universe is not still, and everything inside of you is moving—your heart is beating, your blood is flowing, and your brain is vibrating electrically. For people who have had trouble meditating in a classical way, I suggest the alternative method of Autokinetics.

Autokinetics is a moving meditation that brings forth a natural state of being, a condition of oneness with the ocean of life. But it does so by allowing you to enter into the natural state of movement. Through movement your mind is quieted and freed from its distracting chatter. It empties your inner life by spontaneously acting out that life. This emptying enables you to move with the pulse of life itself and become fully tuned.

Autokinetics introduces you to the most perfect teacher, specifically designed to teach you what you need to know when you need to know it. This teacher is none other than the natural movements of your own body. As you will find out for yourself, when you are moved in a natural way, the guidance that you need for any aspect of your life will come forth naturally.

Dr. Herbert Benson's best-selling book *The Relaxation Response* spelled out what he saw as the four basic elements of meditation: (1) a quiet environment; (2) a word, image, sound, or feeling to focus on; (3) a passive attitude; and (4) a comfortable posture. He and his colleagues at Harvard University proposed a successful technique to bring forth meditative relaxation that involves closing your eyes and counting your breaths for ten to twenty minutes, while maintaining a passive attitude that does not allow distracting thoughts to interfere with your focused state.

Autokinetics brings a new dimension to the meditative tradition and achieves its positive results naturally and effortlessly. When the body moves in an automatic way, it instantly brings forth a state of consciousness that is trancelike and meditative. Here your mind becomes calmed without any difficulty or effort, and the body is both relaxed and energized. Autokinetics celebrates the original goals of ancient and contemporary forms of meditation but offers a swift and effortless way of reaching those goals. It recognizes the healing consequences of a relaxed body, but it goes on to acknowledge that relaxation is a consequence of a tuned body. The concept of tuning suggests that relaxation and energy go hand in hand, not separate from each other. With Autokinetics, our understanding of the relaxation response and the ancient traditions of meditation broadens, enabling us to connect with the even older energy practices of indigenous cultures. With an energy break, your stress is broken down while your whole being is tuned, leaving you both relaxed *and* energized.

How Life Energy Changes Your Diet

Each new weight-loss diet typically professes to have the true remedy for every conceivable issue regarding weight. But despite countless diets and weight control programs and hundreds of clinics for eating disorders, millions of people still have a weight problem. The cultures that are familiar with life energy practices, however, know something that has not yet permeated our culture: there is no such thing as a diet that works for everyone, nor will there ever be. Furthermore, we fail to realize that the problem usually has less to do with what we are eating than with what state of energy we are in. Energy determines good health, and if you have enough of the universal life force, then you are better able to metabolize what you eat and turn it into energy rather than deposit it as excess calories and cellulite.

The oldest way to achieve weight control is to increase your life force. The Asian approach to diet emphasizes energy and recognizes that each person must relate to eating in a flexible way. This means that your diet will always be changing, shifting with your ongoing needs and demands. This is one of the oldest tenets of Chinese medicine.

When you use Autokinetics and get into the daily practice of taking energy breaks that bring the life force into your body, you begin to bring forth new ways of managing your eating behavior. As you learn to tune yourself, one of the things that happens is that you become more sensitive to hearing the call of your own body for certain foods. Rather than being a robotic-like victim of bad eating habits, you start to listen to what your body wants to eat, both in terms of quality and quantity.

Sabotage Your Bad Eating Habits   I often suggest that my clients use Autokinetics in combination with Zenlike dietary interventions. I never tell them what to eat or what to avoid eating. Instead, I suggest unusual ways to interrupt their eating habits. I once suggested to a client who was struggling with weight control that he spend the next week trying to gain exactly one pound. I told him that since his problem was one of "control," finding out how to accurately gain one pound, no more and no less, should teach him something important. He gained that pound and went on to lose the thirty pounds he wanted to drop. Since he had come to me with a well-developed habit of eating too much, I drew on this as a resource and arranged for him to have a successful experience with control rather than to continue being defeated in his customary efforts to conquer his overeating. Once he had some success with control, he was on his way to his desired weight.

Anything that can distract, sabotage, interrupt, or trick you out of a mindless eating habit will help free your mind to listen to what your body wants to eat. The problem is not that you want the wrong things, but that you are simply following a stuck eating habit. You eat that extra snack because it's a habit that blocks you from hearing what your body really wants. It is your body's wisdom that must take over your eating, not the habits of your mind, whether they come from old eating patterns or from what you have just read in a new diet book.

The directives I give are designed to bring forth surprising moments, often humorous or absurd, and provide an opening for a change to take place. This change involves moving the habit out of the way so you can hear what your body is trying to say. Bad eating habits are like having too much wax in your ear, making it impossible to hear what is being spoken. The trick to initiating a good relationship with food is to first clean out the wax so you can hear what your body wants to eat.

The Straw That Broke the Habit's Back   For instance, I saw a young salesman from Memphis who believed he couldn't stop having soft drinks and junk food snacks throughout the day. He was on the road quite often because his job required that he visit different companies. Before driving to his next appointment, he would fill a sack with soft drinks and junk food and drink and eat while he drove. He felt that he was "stuffing his face," to use his words, and he believed that he wasn't even very hungry when he did it. I suggested that he try a little experiment, which would introduce him to a different way of getting a lot of stuff into his mouth. I asked him to do this each time before driving to his next business appointment. He was asked to drink a glass of his favorite beverage with as many straws as he could. The next day he was instructed to drink the same beverage, but this time with one less straw. Each day on the job he was told to repeat this until he had no straws left.

To his great surprise, getting all of those straws into his mouth and then eliminating one at a time was enough to short-circuit his bad habit of stuffing himself with junk food and soft drinks. When he asked me why he was now free of his old habit, I said he always had known that he didn't really want to do it in the first place, or else he wouldn't have sought help. Furthermore, I reminded him that since he knew that he was trying to get unstuck from a bad habit, all we did was throw a monkey wrench into his machinery. With the straw exercise, he was able to stuff his face, but the removal of one straw at a time helped wean him away from his bad habit. Finally, as we were able to humorously reflect on his situation, he eventually got to that last straw, the straw that broke the habit's back. He was now free to get on with his life without being terrorized by this habit—it no longer had a grip on him.

When he cleared away this old habit, I asked him to use Autokinetics as a way of increasing the volume of his body's inner voice. I suggested that he ask the flow of life energy to awaken his inner hearing and to speak loudly enough for him to hear whatever it had to say about eating. With energy breaks, he was able to learn how to eat healthier foods and to enjoy eating in a way he had never known before.

There's Always a Choice　In Seattle, I saw a mother of three young children who ran a day care center in her own home. She believed that she was unable to stop eating: "If it's on the table, I'll eat it, even if I don't want it." She was completely convinced that she was unable to say no to food, and she could not remember a single time in recent history when she had not eaten everything she could get her fork into. I suggested that what was needed to help her become free of this bondage to food was a startling experience—*not* eating all the food that was present during a meal. The experience had to be unusual, I argued, because she needed to be jolted into the realization that it was possible for her not to eat everything that was near her fork.

This is what we arranged for her to do. After an energy break, she went to her kitchen, stood on top of a small stepladder, and ate a meal she had placed on top of her refrigerator. With each bite she took, she said out loud, "I'm really not eating everything beneath my fork." When she did this, she burst into laughter, realizing that she really wasn't eating what was in the refrigerator underneath her plate and fork. She was flooded with the absurdity of her belief and situation, and this was enough to give her a new outlook on eating and a new relationship with eating. Whenever she felt tempted to eat something that she really didn't want, she would think of herself eating that meal on top of her refrigerator, and bring forth a chuckle, an inner tickle that disrupted the influence of that old habit of overeating.

Habits can become such a powerful influence over our lives that we are tempted to believe we have lost the ability to make a choice. This was certainly true for one of my clients, who believed that she could not make a wise choice for herself when she was eating. This applied both to what she chose to eat and to how much of it she ate. I designed a very simple procedure for her that quickly brought her back to her senses, enabling her to fully know that she was always free to make the right choice. She was told to place a brick and a tissue in front of her plate before every evening meal. When she sat down to eat, she was to keep looking at the brick and tissue and say to herself, "It's simply a choice." She knew that whether she ate heavily or lightly was a choice every bit as easy as choosing whether to lift a tissue or a brick. The absurdity of her eating habit was clear when she faced that actual brick and tissue sitting in front of her at her evening meal. As she faced this absurdity, I asked her to move her body and initiate a brief version of Autokinetics, waiting for herself to enter the tuning zone. After she was tuned, she could proceed to eat her meal. This new and unexpected difference in experiencing her meal was enough to free her from the misconception that she couldn't stop eating, and led her to listen to her own inner voice of wisdom.

You're Halfway There One of the ways I have found useful in helping free people from stuck eating habits involves asking them to imagine that only half of their body has the "weight problem." If you have a problem with overeating, try this out for yourself. It makes sense, after all, since the other part of you tries to control your weight and wants to be in good shape. Choose which side you think is the problem—the left side or the right side. If you don't know, follow your intuition. If you're still not sure, ask the person you believe is most intuitive to make the choice. Every time you think about eating too much or taking a bite of a "problem" food, lean your body to the problem side (bend the neck, tilt the head, and so forth). If you say no, then lean back to the balanced position. If you give in, remain tilted for five minutes after you've given in to the problem side. After this position has been held, I suggest that you sit down and do a brief version of the energy break, swaying back and forth until you enter the tuning zone.

Doing this sort of procedure is a powerful way of interrupting the problem eating pattern that you're trying to get free from and puts you in a position to turn on the movements of Autokinetics. By acting as if part of your body is the problem, you introduce the belief that the rest of your body can do something about it. Moving your body from side to side also changes the whole experience of eating the problem food, making it more obvious that this is a ridiculous experience—as ridiculous as eating what you really don't want to eat, simply because of a stupid habit.

One of my favorite cases involved a student at the University of Arizona who had fallen into the bad habit of eating too much in the college cafeteria and was beginning to suffer from being overweight. I simply asked him to arrange his meals so that all of his food was on only half his plate. He was told to keep the other side of the plate empty to remind him of what he didn't have to eat. He continued this way of arranging the food on his plate until he became accustomed to it. At that point he was told to stop doing it. To his surprise, thereafter he never put more on his plate than he needed. This was all it took to free his mind to recognize that he could always make the right choice and that it was an illusion that he was under the spell of a bad eating habit. Indeed, one way out of a bad habit involves bumping it out of office by electing another habit, one that gives you more freedom to make the choice you really want to make. And once you've taken a step away from a bad habit, it's natural to take the next step—allowing the flow of the life force to move through you in such a way that it opens you to hear the wisdom of your own body.

The Energy Solution to Weight Control You may be wondering why anyone would do these odd rituals, but keep in mind that their purpose is to throw a monkey wrench into your eating habits, freeing your mind to listen to the wisdom of your own body. Like the tasks and riddles given by Zen teachers or indigenous shamans and healers, the rituals direct you to go outside of the boundaries of your habitual behavior and to have an experience that throws you into the absurdity of your situation. The predicament we are in has less to do with an eating problem than with a "dumb habit." When we interrupt the way we are glued to these habits, we free ourselves to be in a more natural state of being, one that listens to the resonance of our own body's true needs and desires.

Finding ways to interrupt your problem eating habits is only half the job of getting back on the road to healthy eating and weight control. The other half involves taking energy breaks that bring the life force into your body. This strengthens the body and helps you better metabolize whatever you choose to eat. It also gives more volume to your body's voice, which awaits your listening to and following its directives about what foods you most desire.

If you are struggling with your eating habits and diet, keep these energy insights in mind:

- When making a decision about eating, do a scaled-down version of the energy break; and while your body moves itself toward the tuning zone, ask whether your body really wants that food or whether this is the mindless reaction of a stuck habit.
- If you find yourself caught in a bad habit, become an espionage agent who seeks to infiltrate the habit pattern and disrupt it. Realize that you must escape being a prisoner of this habit. Rather than fighting the entrenched habit directly, which tends to bring forth its resistive forces, trick it by going in the *direction* of the habit and then add something ridiculous or startling to it. This will free you by making the experience as ridiculous and absurd as it really is.
- When you are free from bad eating habits, don't be unnecessarily influenced by diet experts. Enter into the tuned zone and listen first and foremost to the calling of your own body.
- If you take a bite of something and it tastes "off" or not quite right, then don't eat it. There is nothing wrong with changing your mind and deciding not to eat something. You can always choose to pause for a moment, bring about some small body movements so as to move yourself toward the tuning zone, and

then listen to your body speak. When your body doesn't really want something, it is not uncommon for that unwanted food to taste unpleasant or not to live up to the taste you remember.

- On the other hand, when something really tastes wonderful, go after it. But stop when you feel that you have had enough. If you are not sure, wait awhile to see if you are satisfied. Don't get caught in the automatic habit of stuffing yourself. Wait for your body to ask for each bite. If that sweet tooth has a hold on you, go into the tuning zone and pay extra-close attention to what your body really says it wants.

- On a daily basis, tell yourself that you believe in the wisdom of your body. Trust your body, and when you take an energy break, ask its movements to speak to you with more authority. Acknowledge that you will strive to give it the attention it deserves.

- Believe that every food in the world provides nutrition when you enter into the appropriate energy resonance with it, although any one food may not be right for you at any particular moment.

- When you eat, recognize that you are having an energy encounter with life. The life force of another living thing is transferring its energy to you. Think of eating as a special energy event rather than a mundane experience of consumption.

The energy way of life brings you to a table that is free of diet books and weight-control programs. It asks that you stop being controlled by mindless habits and the conflicting instructions of so-called experts. No one can know what is best for you to eat except your own body. It is the perfect dietician for you. Clear your dinner table of all outside distractions and learn how to listen to your own inner expertise. Hand over your diet to your body and allow it to wisely feast upon the energy that life brings to your dining experiences.

Beyond Exercise as You Now Know It

We often encounter two attitudes regarding exercise that do *not* foster the well-being of the body. The first is "hibernation"—the all-too-familiar attitude of the couch potato. This inactivity sometimes causes us to take up the second attitude, and we exercise till we drop—hence the proliferation of personal trainers and health clubs. The almost fanatical zeal with which aerobics evangelists, thigh-master priestesses, and technoexercise gurus spread their word inspires many of us to plunge headfirst into the latest exercise craze.

We often hear that our contemporary health problems stem from lack of exercise, but we rarely encounter the warning that it is not good for us to exercise too much. However, when you become dedicated to taking energy breaks—that is, the daily practice of Autokinetics—you find a simple solution to the issue of exercise and physical fitness. You realize that what is most important is for your body to move naturally, and that you should not always force it to do something unnatural or too fatiguing. From this perspective, the wisest exercise for everyday vitality involves stretching and moving in the ways that Autokinetics brings forth. Of course, if you have a passion for a sport, then by all means go out and play it, but do so effortlessly and naturally.

Dr. Robert Fulford laments the shape the body gets into when we exercise too much. In the years of his private practice he found too many tight bodies that were completely out of whack, having strayed far from the naturally loose form we were designed to embody. He mentions one of his colleagues in Boston, another osteopath, who keeps a small sandbag in his office, ready to hit overly muscled patients with it in order to help loosen them up.

It is no accident that cultures around the world that nurture a practice of circulating the life force do not promote the kind of exercise and physical fitness we promote. Like the Asian view of diet, the life energy perspective on exercise seeks movements that enhance the life force in our bodies. In China, millions of people engage in the daily practice of tai chi or chi gong, ways of making gentle and natural movements. Unlike modern calisthethetics and strenuous exercise regimes that drain us of energy, these ancient practices move more energy into our body. They understand how too much unnatural movement and exercise can be harmful.

Do Less   Dr. Fulford suggests in *Dr. Fulford's Touch of Life* that we are better off stretching ten minutes a day than attending four aerobic exercise classes a week. The kind of simple stretching that moves naturally with your breathing and the flow of the life force results in optimal body tone, which truly promotes lifelong vitality.

If you are too sedentary, then introduce some gentle stretching into your life. On the other hand, if you are overinvolved in physical conditioning, then I suggest that you consider slowing down and substituting some simple stretching movements. Do not stop overnight. This may be too strong a shock to your body, and it may make you prone to having an accident. Gently withdraw from spending too much time in the gym or in the exercise class. If strenuous activity gives you a natural high, then treat yourself to it with the same kind of moderation that should be used in eating desserts. A little dose every once in a while is a delightful treat, but too much of a good thing is not wise. I know this may sound like shocking advice, but it's the same recommendation you would get anywhere in the world from someone who is working and living with an understanding of the universal life force.

The One-Minute Fitness Program   I worked with a middle-aged man who had never done much exercise, but now wanted to do whatever would help him maintain his health. After reading many self-help books and attending introductions to various health spas and exercise programs, he listened to what I had to say about Autokinetics. He began practicing it on a daily basis and then came up with his own fitness program. He decided to exercise for no longer than one minute at a time. He had heard of the "one-minute manager" and decided to develop a one-minute fitness program. During the course of his workday he set aside the first minute of each hour to do what he called his "fitness version" of Autokinetics. He would excuse himself from a meeting, or go for a drink of water, and allow his body to fall into a natural rhythm of movement, allowing every limb to be stretched and moved. He did this eight times a day, one minute for every hour he was at work. To his delight he found that after doing this for several months, he could feel a change in his body. He felt more fit and had more energy and strength in his muscles. To this day he never exercises more than one minute at a time but does exercise every hour of his workday.

The daily practice of Autokinetics naturally brings stretching movements into your daily life. These exercises do not consume a lot of energy, but they awaken and circulate energy within your body. As you practice this effortless method, you will find that certain changes take place in your internal organs and muscles. This happens because your whole being is exercised and brought into a more dynamic flow with life itself.

The Kinetic Zone   Recall how a trancelike state comes over you when you move into the final step of Autokinetics. This fall into your natural movements takes you toward being "in the zone"—the "zone" athletes refer to when they are completely tuned to playing their sport. One of my clients reported to me that when she is completely absorbed in Autokinetics, something amazing takes place. She experiences the life energy as if she were in a body of water, and her movements become the same as if she were actually swimming through this water.

Athletes who use Autokinetics become more skilled in feeling the life force around them. I encourage them to bring this new sense of the life force into their game plan, and they try to fall into the movements of their sport in an automatic and natural way. I invite them to visualize what I call the *kinetic zone,* a field of energy that, like a motion picture, is always moving its shape and pattern. They then move to seeing each motion of the body in an athletic activity as being held by this changing energy field, so that throwing a football, for example, is seen as a pattern that holds the entire event. If athletes get into sync with this pattern, all they have to do is step into it—and all of the action will then take place without effort. These athletes feel like children sliding down a big slide in a playground. They do nothing except allow the body to go along for the ride.

You don't have to be an athlete to benefit from this process of visualization. Any physical work or exercise can be done in this way. If you are doing something as simple as moving a heavy object, pause for a moment to visualize a force field that connects your body with the weight. Imagine that when you step into this field of energy and align yourself with it in a natural way, the object can be lifted with as little effort as is possible. Doing this—something that ancient Asian practitioners of life energy have always done—will help prevent back injury and will give you an opportunity to practice being more in tune with the life force.

A senior tennis player from San Diego started working with Autokinetics and used its ideas to guide her daily routine of stretching exercises. Before each exercise she would close her eyes and imagine an energy field around the particular movement she wanted to perform. After she created that image, she would start the stretching movement, believing that the field of energy was actually moving her. This visualization helped her do the exercise with little effort or strain. Each movement of each exercise, from bending over to standing on her toes, was done with the belief that she was entering into an energy field that allowed the movement to take place without any effort on her part. With the three-step technique of Autokinetics she learned to make the kind of natural movements in her exercise program that brought more energy into her daily life.

This way of natural movement is similar to that of the ancient Japanese tradition of Zen archery. In this practice, in his mind's eye, the archer becomes inseparable from the target, the bow, and the arrow, so that the release of the arrow and its entry into the bull's-eye involve no luck and no skill but make up an automatic movement taking place within a natural pattern—where all is connected, from the beginning of the act (before releasing the arrow) all the way to the conclusion (the arrow stuck in the center of the target). This is an ancient secret that explains the high performance levels achieved by masters of a sport or art. They do not necessarily concentrate or work any harder than anyone else or practice in any special way to achieve their level of expertise. They have found a way to jump into the pattern that carries their body through the perfect motions required for the desired outcome.

Effortless Exercise   The natural way to exercise invites you to do less in order to get more. You aim to still your strained efforts to be physically fit in order to be energetically moved by life. In this movement you become the natural shape that is healthiest for you.

When you change your philosophy and practice of exercise to the natural energy way, you will find that it brings a complete redefinition of what you think exercise is all about. As you walk through each day, the various activities that come to you will be seen as opportunities to exercise the movement of the life force. You can immediately start getting ready for this change in your daily outlook by seeing the movements of each day as an invitation to do some Autokinetics. For example, when you are out shopping, think of using your energy, rather than your muscles, to lift and carry. And when you are on the phone, using a computer, or sitting in a chair, think about how you can move the life force into your body, whether it be through swaying back and forth or wiggling your fingers. Simply thinking about this goal will help trigger your body to alter your posture or move yourself to facilitate the flow of revitalizing energy. Meet every activity in your life—driving to work, watching television, or preparing the evening meal—as an opportunity to exercise the natural movements that bring more life into your daily experiences.

The energy approach to exercise is the most natural way to take care of your physical body. Keep these tips in mind when you consider changing your exercises to be more in tune with the life force:

- Say no to excessive physical strain and avoid the energy drain. Move naturally with the flow of your physical movements and receive an energy charge.
- What counts is not the amount of exercise you perform but the quality of naturalness in your movements.

- Move from expending energy in your exercise to resonating with energy. In other words, flow with the physical movements in a way that brings you into the tuning zone, the place where you are energized and vitalized.
- A minute a day of natural movement may do more for your well-being than marathons and strenuous workouts.
- The natural way of exercise always feels good. It is comforting and delightful, not uncomfortable or painful. If an exercise hurts, stop doing it.
- The amount of physical stress your body can safely handle depends on how naturally you are able to move yourself.
- Dance, the movement of your body to rhythm, is really the only exercise. All sports are dances, that is, orchestrated movements with their own unique rhythms and timing. Whether you are playing basketball, tennis, or soccer, realize that it is a dance, and that what holds true for the dance floor also holds true for the sports arena.

The energy way of life sees every movement that you take as an opportunity for energizing yourself. Exercise should not be an activity that you separate from the rest of your life. It should be integrated within the whole of your life. Walking, running, jumping, sitting, breathing, lifting an arm, curling a toe, wiggling a finger are the movements of our daily physical exercise. Bring all of these movements into the rhythms that make them more natural and more energizing. If a sport brings pleasure to you, then by all means do it if you can. Do so with the spirit of play and know that a sport, or a particular physical exercise, offers its highest rewards to those who fall into the zone, the place where your movements are most naturally perfect and most naturally energizing to your whole life.

Finding Effective Ways to Solve Your Problems

One of the most amazing outcomes of Autokinetics is how it can bring forth new and effective solutions to the difficulties and challenges of your life. Tune in to the universal life force whenever you have a problem that needs to be solved. This is done by momentarily focusing on your problem before you start the natural movements of Autokinetics. As you sit and prepare to enter into these movements, talk to yourself and simply state, with no worry or overconcern, what you would like help with. Then fall into an energy break, knowing that it may bring forth a new idea, tactic, or suggestion for how to deal with your situation. You can make this kind of request for anything that you want help with in your life, including your diet, exercise, self-healing, personal development, and specific everyday problems.

Nurture Energy, Forget Words   Do not indulge in overanalyzing any difficulty in your life. Make an agreement with yourself that the things that bother and disturb you will be dealt with when you practice Autokinetics. The less you think about the problem and the more you hand it over to the natural flow of the life force, the more likely the solution you are searching for will appear. An ancient Taoist philosopher, Chang San-feng, put it this way: "Nurture energy, forget words, and guard it." In other words, nurture your energy instead of using words to figure it out. This applies to every imaginable problem you may encounter—job difficulties, personal struggles, life crises, relationship issues, and existential dilemmas. Take them to your practice and allow them to be bathed and washed in the flow of the life force. In this process, a creative solution may be born.

The solution may come to you in various ways. You may see, hear, or feel it during the session itself; or you may wake up in the middle of the night after a dream that gives you specific advice; or you may have a sudden, spontaneous realization of such a dream the following day. Trust that life will answer your questions and do not become attached to a form in which you expect the answer to come to you. An answer may be direct or indirect, literal or metaphorical, heard or seen, known logically or felt viscerally. When you turn over your personal issues to the whole of life, wait patiently for the wisdom of life to move you forward in its own way.

Like the energy approach to dieting, effective problem solving requires that you accomplish two things. First, you must find a way to quiet those habits that make it impossible for you to hear your inner guidance and wisdom. In other words, stop the type of ineffective strategies you've been trying. If they had worked, you wouldn't now be concerned about what should be done. One way to stop your ineffective habits is to engage in an uncommon task or activity that is designed to distract you and short-circuit the way you typically do things. When your mind is freed from its stuck habits and its noisy thinking is quieted, then you become more ready for the second thing you must do to get an effective solution. Now you are prepared to take an energy break and tap into the life force, mobilizing it to bring you a new and effective solution. This is what you do when you sit down and practice Autokinetics.

Following are examples of some of the tasks used by clients who were stuck in their everyday difficulties. These tasks were given to still their ineffective habits, preparing them to use Autokinetics successfully as a means of consulting with their own inner resources.

Put That Worrying to Work   One of my clients was an elementary school teacher from Kansas City, Missouri, who couldn't stop worrying. She worried about her job, her children, her parents, and her own health. After a year of counseling, her worrying hadn't stopped. She was then referred to me, and I suggested that she see if she could stop worrying about her worrying. I immediately invited her to try something that might help put her mind at ease. She was told to purchase a children's bank from a toy store and then bring it home and put it in an obvious place, such as the top of her television set. Every time she caught herself worrying for longer than a minute, she was to put a quarter in the bank. She promised to be honest and feed the bank whenever she worried too much. When the bank was full, she agreed to donate the money to a worthy organization. I explained that she could now stop worrying about her worries because she had put her worrying to work. It would now help others when she was unable to help herself.

The young schoolteacher experienced firsthand how her worries could be transformed into serving a positive outcome, and in so doing she found that she was not totally helpless. She could tame her worrying rather than be frightened and overpowered by it. Once she was able to stop worrying about her worries, she was able to achieve more freedom from her problem.

This shift enabled her to enter more confidently into Autokinetics, with a request for something else she could do when a worry came her way. During one of her energy breaks she daydreamed a new solution. She saw herself purchasing a small rug that could be rolled up and hidden in a place undisturbed by others. When she found herself worrying too much, she would pull out the rug and spread it on the floor. She would then take off her shoes and socks and stand on the rug. As she did this she would ask her mind to let go of any worry that was in her head, and she would allow gravity to pull each worry to the bottom of her feet. As her worries began moving toward the ground, she would wiggle her toes, pretending that this was caused by the worries' entering them. She would wiggle her toes for at least ten seconds and would then stomp her feet on the mat so that she could completely shake out those worries. When she vigorously completed this task, she would pick up the rug, take it outside and shake it—to shake out her worries. Then she would roll up the rug and give it a rest so that it would be ready should she need to use it again.

The schoolteacher did exactly what she saw herself doing in her daydream and found that it was an effective solution for handling her worries. You, too, can follow her example and that of numerous others who have sat down to energize themselves with Autokinetics while asking for a solution to one of their life problems. When you do so, your creative imagination and inner resources will be mobilized by the flow of the life force to give birth to an idea that can help you.

A florist in San Francisco who had trouble with worrying sat down to energize herself and came up with this creative solution. Not only did her advice work for her own situation; it has also worked for others who suffer from worrying too much. Here's the answer that came to her in her energy break:

Find another person who worries as much as you. For one week, swap your worries. Each of you must make a list of your top worries and give it to the other person. Be sincere in your efforts to worry daily about the other person's concerns. You may find that learning to worry about someone else's worries helps free you from your own.

The florist's solution to worrying involves finding another person who has the same problem. Rather than sit around and complain about the shared problem, her advice is to put each person to work handling the problem of the other person. Now, when she herself takes an energy break, she does so with a request for solutions for the other person's worrying. Moving with the problem, rather than fighting it or complaining about it, has helped her move forward. The key here is that she has found a way to use her problem as a resource—in this case, a resource for another person—and this has helped her become free from the incapacitating hold of worrying over her daily life.

Energize a New Self-Image   I once met a graduate student who was having difficulty with his self-image. He thought that no one could be attracted to him as a friend. As a means of helping him block this bad attitude about himself, I asked if he knew a child who looked up to him. He quickly acknowledged that his nephew was his greatest fan. I then suggested that he ask his nephew do him the favor of drawing a picture of him. He was to provide the child with whatever crayons or watercolors were needed to accomplish the task. I told him that it was very important that he never see this picture. He was to receive it in a sealed envelope and then put the envelope into his pillow. I advised him to take his pillow to someone who could sew; that person would open the pillow, place the envelope in it, and sew it back up. When this was completed, he was told to periodically rest his head on this pillow, giving some consideration to how he thought he was seen by his nephew.

This task planted a positive seed in his mind. I advised him to lay his head on that pillow for a few minutes before he took an energy break so that this would bring him into touch with the favorable way his nephew saw him. Seeing himself through his nephew's eyes helped unlock him from the negative views he feared others had of him. This gave him a fresh resource to work with, and when he was regularly energized by the life force, it was sufficient to stimulate the building of a whole new self-image, one filled with confidence and self-assurance.

Getting Motivated   There are many people who not only suffer from a
poor self-image but lack the confidence they believe they need to be
successful. I often tell these people to go to a place where a "motiva-
tional expert" is offering a speech or workshop on motivation. I in-
struct them to not attend the workshop, but instead, wait until there is
a lunch break and, with a notebook, talk to at least ten people who are
in attendance. I tell them to ask each person to give one sentence that
summarizes the most important thing he or she learned about being
motivated; to write these sentences down; and, over the next ten days,
to give one day to considering each sentence. They carry the sentence
around all day and think about all the different ways they could communicate the same idea. After they've lived with each statement, they
write their own overall sentence that represents what they think is
most important about being motivated.

This task moves you to go on a search for the clues that can help
you find your own answer to the problem of motivation. When you finally come up with your individualized one-sentence answer, I suggest that you hold this sentence in your mind whenever you take an
energy break. When you hold this answer in your mind as the life
force surges through you, it helps awaken your own motivation. Your
idea about motivation is energized by the practice, and you feel more
ready to go after the success you desire.

Releasing Fear   Sometimes people get stuck in unnecessary fear, but
this, too, can be short-circuited by a simple task. Years ago, I worked
with a war veteran who was plagued with inappropriate fear. I advised
him to literally blow it up. I instructed him to put two teaspoonsful of
Rice Krispies in a small bowl, stare into the bowl, and imagine
projecting his fear onto the cereal, as if he had a special kind of
thought power. He was instructed to hold the bowl and shake the

cereal around as if he were able to transmit the vibrations of fear into the cereal. He was then to put the cereal in a pair of his shoes—one teaspoon for each foot—and proceed to take a fifteen-minute walk. I asked him to pay attention to feeling the fearful Rice Krispies become pulverized as he walked on top of them, and to imagine the crunchy sounds that were being made. After his walk, I told him to empty the Rice Krispies into his hand and complete the job of pulverizing them, turning them into a powder. He was instructed to put the powder on a piece of tissue paper, wrap it up, and pretend that it was a bomb—a "fear bomb." He was instructed to take his bomb to a safe place and ignite it, carefully listening to hear whether it exploded. I asked him to determine the power of his fear by the loudness of the explosion.

When he carried out this assignment, he experienced the absurdity of his fear, and this was enough to let him release it. When he subsequently took an energy break, he found he could bring forth the memory of that "fear bomb," remembering the sense of absurdity that rushed through him when he actually ignited it. When the life force moved through him, bringing a realization of the absurd way in which he had been stuck, it became a powerful means of washing away his inappropriate terror and panic.

Planting Your Solution   I often ask people to choose one word that best describes what they learned when they did an absurd task. When they come up with a word, I ask them to repeat it over and over again during several energy breaks. If you do this, it will help plant in your mind the seed of what you learned. When the life force moves through you, it will plant and germinate this idea deep within you and allow other, related ideas, learning, answers, and advice to sprout into your awareness.

I once worked with some court-assigned adult probation cases dealing with issues of handling anger. I sometimes advised these clients to choose one finger and designate it as their "finger of anger." I suggested that whenever they became angry, they flutter this finger in a rapid vibratory movement. They were advised to imagine that the vibration was the "pulse" of their anger. They were to keep vibrating the angry finger until they detected their anger starting to dissipate.

Sometimes it's hard even for me to believe that such a simple task is enough to derail a habit, particularly when it involves a problem as serious as bouts of wild anger. Yet I have seen, time and time again, that the best way out of a stuck problem is to trip it while it is happening or about to happen. Don't try to block it, but stick your leg out in front of it and watch it trip over itself. When you get a sense of how little it actually takes to get unstuck from a habitual problem, you can take an energy break and request that your imagination cook up a creative way of tripping yourself out of whatever mess you happen to be stuck in.

Wave Good-Bye to Your Troubles   There is an ancient yoga technique of clearing the mind that involves staring at one point on a wall while waving your hand back and forth in front of your eyes, like the windshield wiper of a car. When this is done for an extended period of time, there is a feeling that old problems and worries are being wiped away, leaving room in your mind for a fresh beginning. The modern equivalent of this technique is called "eye movement desensitization and reprocessing" (EMDR) and was developed by a clinical psychologist, Dr. Francine Shapiro. Over 1 million clients have been treated with this method, which suggests that people are released from the hold of a past traumatic experience by simply getting them to think of the problem while their eyes move back and forth as they watch a therapist wave his or her hand.

I believe that this approach is successful because of the simple eye movement it initiates. However, from the perspective of Autokinetics it works only with the tip of the iceberg. Underneath the movement of eyeballs is a body that also wants to move and fall into an improvised rhythm. When this takes place, it does more than wipe your mental slate clean. It invites your own creative processes to be energized by the life force and leads you to new ideas for moving your life forward. I invite you to aim for more than a clearing of your emotions and problematic mental habits. Set a higher mark: transforming your irritations, difficulties, problems, and suffering as a means of propelling you to a more rewarding and vibrant life.

Await the tasks that promise to take you into an uncommon experience of the problem that concerns you, whether it be fear, motivation, worrying, dieting, or whatever. Such a task is so different from your typical habits of action and contemplation that it makes an opening through which new possibilities can enter. Doing this kind of task also prepares you to receive even more answers and benefits from Autokinetics. When you have a problem that you're struggling with, do something uncommon and creatively different with it for at least a week or two and ask for further help during your energy break. When this is done, a larger opening is made for more creative solutions to pour forth naturally.

The energy way of finding solutions to everyday problems can be summarized with these guidelines:

- If the problem has repeated itself three times, consider it a habit. If it's not a habit, it usually will go away on its own.
- When you're up against a habit, remind yourself that any resistance to it will probably strengthen it. Don't fight the habit, but find a way to trick it. The best way to trick yourself out of a habit

is to trip yourself over it. Do this by accepting the habit and using it in a way that carries it toward absurdity, either by finding a way in which it can be a resource for something or someone else or by allowing it to move you into having a full-blown experience of the ridiculousness of your situation.

• Use Autokinetics to ask for habit-busting tasks. In the trance-like tuning zone, it is most likely that your creative mind can come up with some ideas and tasks—or clues for ideas and tasks—that you can try.

• Realize that the best advice for dealing with your difficulty will come from the energy of life itself. When you have the life force pulsing through your creative mind, you are maximizing the odds that a well-designed solution will be found. Not only will the wave of the life force help wash away your old problems; it will bring in new experiences and resources.

Like everything else that happens to you in life, problems are another opportunity for you to be moved by the energy that they naturally carry. Allow the energy of everyday difficulties, problems, dilemmas, and challenges to move you into Autokinetics with a request for creative guidance, the kind of advice that frees you from fighting your situation and invites you to join with life as a coconspirator. Explore the many ways that a problem can be tricked into becoming a solution, a resource, even an inspiration for your future.

Awakening Your Personal Creativity

As you move into the charged life, you will develop a whole new outlook on the subject of creativity. You will discover firsthand how simply taking an energy break not only brings forth the life force but turns on your inner creative juices. When the life force is awakened, creativity is present. As energy moves through you, so will the natural ability to have more creative expression. As you practice Autokinetics, your day-to-day life will be touched with newfound creativity.

Whether you ask for a solution to a difficulty or request advice for how your life should progress or inquire about creative ideas for a special project, do this during the time when you are flowing with the life force so as to bring more creative inspiration into the guidance of your life. Be attentive to the ways in which you feel drawn to express yourself. Do you want to take on a special project, begin keeping a journal, start a new way of cooking, organize a singing group, or invent a new way of collecting humorous sayings? Be on the lookout for detecting a new hunger and a new desire to create.

Bring more creative expression into your life as a means of facilitating the flow of the energizing, healing life force. I am aware of people who have overcome an illness by simply getting lost in a creative project. The well-known novelist Anthony Burgess was once so sick that his doctor gave him little time to live. He immediately decided to make the best use of his time and went off and lost himself in a major writing project. To his doctor's great surprise, he survived and flourished.

When Norman Cousins, another literary figure, decided to treat a life-threatening illness with heavy doses of humor, it may have been his complete immersion in this project as much as his laughter that led to his cure. Similarly, Dr. Bernie Siegel has found that people who survive a critical illness are often those who have not given up on life. They have made their own survival a major creative project, reading every book they could get their hands on, trying various treatments, and listening to their own inner voice as to what they might try next. Immersion in a creative project is a way of activating the flow of the universal life process.

Start a Truly Creative Project   Do not wait until you are sick to throw yourself into a creative project. Do so now and discover how it brings even more energy and vitality into your everyday life. During your practice of Autokinetics, make a simple, clear request for guidance in the expression of your inborn creativity. If you haven't yet discovered your own unique way of being creative, then ask that you be led to it. If you know what kind of creative expression stirs your soul, then ask for how it is to be directed. I worked with a well-known Jungian therapist in St. Paul, Minnesota, who found that the movement of life energy in her body awakened the desire to write a novel. Another client, an architect in New York City, found that the movements brought an inspiration to make pottery.

When you receive an intuition, a well-formed image, or an abstract clue that is related to your personal creativity, whether it be during an energy break or after, follow up on it immediately. For example, let us say that in the course of your practice you find yourself immersed in contemplative reflection about a certain flower. If this happens, you should plan to go out immediately following the exercise, and take some action that involves this flower. Perhaps you would purchase the flower, grow it, draw it, read about it, or write a poem about it. Do anything with it that comes to your mind and stirs your curiosity, passion, and interest. In such an action you activate and feed your creative processes and move them to be more powerfully present in your life.

The Flying Fox   I was working with a physician from St. Paul, and in the course of conducting the Autokinetics technique we brought up the subject of a flying fox. Since the fox had spontaneously flown into our conversation, I thought it would be a good idea to have its image near the place where the physician dreamed—that is, his bedroom.

With my encouragement, he read what he could about this creature and then cut out a picture of the animal so he could hang it from one corner of his bedroom ceiling. The following week, after a highly charged energy break, he remembered that one of the most emotional experiences of his childhood was discovering a dead bat in the family water tank. At that time, he became so curious about the bat that he carefully dissected it and was amazed to find out how part of its structure was like that of a human being. He became so enraptured by the bat that his mother was quite astonished, and she took the time to have a special talk with him about it. This was, as he put it, one of the key impressions of his childhood.

When he realized that the flying fox was actually a bat and began to associate the relationship between this creature and the childhood incident, a surge of energized mystery began to flow in our conversation. As we wondered how the presence of that flying fox in his bedroom could affect him, he remembered something unusual about his dreams: almost all of them had to do with a cave. Furthermore, he realized that he did most of his dreaming in his vacation cabin, which happened to be an underground structure built beneath the earth, like a cave. With these insights, his creative imagination and his desire to express himself creatively came alive. He began sketching images of bats and writing short stories, and this opened him to a creative journey that brought more mystery, wonder, and enchantment into his everyday life. The symbolic content of these events and the words that might be used to explain their meaning were less important than the creative energy that his experiences had inspired.

Dream Journey   The gymnast who came to me with a knee problem also found that the flow of the life force was inseparable from the flow of her creative processes. After working in an Autokinetics session, we started talking about a special box that her grandmother had once given her. I told her to be on the lookout for a dream in which she might encounter this box. The very next night she dreamed of the box and heard a voice tell her to open it. She did, and found that it held a tiny snake, all coiled up. This didn't frighten her, but it made her curious. I told her that cultures throughout the world depict the snake as a symbol of the life force.

I asked her to keep track of her dreams for the following week and to choose one word for each dream that would best represent the meaning it held. For the dream she had just had, she chose the word "snake." When she returned for her next session, she was delighted to report that she had experienced three powerful dreams.

The first dream involved a frightening criminal entering her house. She hid in the closet and covered herself with a pile of clothes. When the intruder opened the closet door and lifted off the clothes, he looked at her and said, "There is no one here." He then left, and she was not harmed in any way. The word for that dream was "fear," and we discussed how the last three years of her life had been filled with the fear that she would never be able to perform a gymnastic routine again. For three years, she had sought help in numerous forms, but she had not competed in a single competition. In this dream, however, she faced fear, and it did not come in. She was not available for fear to enter.

The second night she dreamed of being near the edge of a canyon. There she turned into a cloud and was able to fly over the canyon, and over a forest that was right next to it. Her word for that dream was "cloud," and it captured her feeling of being weightless and able to fly without effort.

In the third dream she had that week, she saw herself in a gymnastic competition performing her routine with absolute perfection.

She chose the words "desired reality" to capture the essence of that dream and noted that she experienced complete ecstasy in it.

She then took the words that she had chosen for her dreams and constructed a sentence with them that would capture what she had learned from her daily practice of Autokinetics. The sentence that she came up with was this: "When you see the coiled *snake*, know that some will see *fear*, while you will see the secret to life, the life force and energy that turns you into a weightless *cloud* and effortlessly moves you to your *desired reality.*" She decided to focus on this sentence whenever she was about to perform her gymnastic routine. The very next evening she performed for the first time in three years. She placed in two of her events and led her team to first place.

I suggest that you go through each day and week as a hunter who tracks down moments that hold some inspiration for your creative development. When you hear a line from a poem that moves you, or see a beautiful scene that charges your heart, or smell a fragrance that lifts your spirit, pause to write down a brief description of the experience, and then carry with you the memory of this brief moment of inspiration. Take it to your next energy break and read it out loud before you do the practice. See this as a way of planting your session with the inspirational seeds that flow through your everyday life. As the life force moves its energy over these acorns of inspiration, they may germinate and mature into future episodes of creative expression. In this way you can use Autokinetics to help grow your own garden of creativity and thereby bring more beauty into your life.

I invite you to enter into the life force with the full awareness that it will bring with it the desire for, and the voice of, your creative expression. Open yourself to the ways it will connect you with your creative imagination, whether it be from your night dreams or daydreams. Pay attention to your charged intuitions and empower them to be brought into the actions of your everyday life. In this way you will find your own way of bringing the joys and delights of creative expression into the world.

Skinship with Others: The Art of Revitalizing Your Intimate Relationships by Touching

Autokinetics provides a powerful way of inspiring your personal and intimate relationships through its use of energized touch and movement. Each of us is born with a desire for *skinship* with others— a desire to touch and be touched—for it is the experience of skin contact that helps awaken, heal, and move us to the fullest realization of life. But in a social climate that rightly fears sexually transmitted disease and charges of sexual misconduct, we face the unfortunate consequences of "touch phobia" and "touch illiteracy." We too often fear the engagement of skin and find that touch is often interpreted as illicit sexuality.

Autokinetics calls for a more hopeful and rewarding direction for touch. It invites us to introduce ourselves to the widest possible range of sensual and illuminating possibilities that touch presents, both inside and outside the bedroom, and pay more respect to the fact that loving, energized touch is necessary for our health and well-being.

The natural movements, energetic expression, and inner teaching that come from practicing Autokinetics call you to touch in a safe and responsible way, without unnecessarily limiting your passionate desire for sensual awareness and exploration. Autokinetics can open the door to a creative eroticism, defining and encouraging a sacred understanding and practice of touch.

We long for the inspired touching that energizes us to feel and express the tender warmth and luminous glow of love, whether this touching comes from the tactile contact of a lover's caress, the music of sensuous poetry, or the scent of a lilac in spring. We touch and are touched not only with our skin but also with what is shown, smelled, tasted, and imagined. Unless we are energetically and heartfully touched in these ways, life too easily becomes a tiresome set of routines, wearing us down and making us despondent about the past, present, and future. We have become overloaded with self-help catchphrases, but short on the kind of touching that can inspire and transform our emotional and relational lives.

Expanding Your Vocabulary of Touch As you practice Autokinetics, see it as a tuning and cleansing of all of your senses. Follow your practice with an experience that brings you some sensory delight. Read a poem, listen to some music, touch the earth, smell a special aroma, look at a beautiful work of art, write a letter, or take a walk in a natural setting. Notice how much more alive you feel when you are tuned and how life is able to touch your senses more dramatically.

Through touch, the energy of life can also flow between people. The tingling of energy that stirs us to be more fully alive has historically been called *eros,* defined not only as the energy of life and sexuality, but more generally as the organic impulse toward relationship and wholeness, the force that links people together through the desire for love—the complete, boundless state of unity.

Touch in Family Life There are many opportunities for touching in everyday family life. We may comb each other's hair, scratch each other's backs, and tickle one another. Families who energize themselves with the life force will find many ways of touching one another and will find touching a natural way to alleviate the stress and irritations that arise in their daily work, as well as an everyday practice of expressing their affection for one another.

Touch your family members or intimate partners with the kind of improvisational touch that you practice on yourself in Autokinetics. Give them an improvisational massage by letting your fingers and hands freely move over them. Do this while sending loving energy toward them. Get out of the habit of sitting passively with one another in the evenings. If your family watches television together, then do so while touching and rubbing one another and allowing the life force to move through the whole family.

Touch in Daily Life   Each day presents us with numerous opportunities to touch others outside the family. There we may exercise various choreographies of handshaking, backslapping, pats on the back, and hugging that make up our daily skinship. Through Autokinetics you learn to energize this tactile contact in a way that brings forth more positive resonances in your daily interactions. For instance, when you shake someone's hand, you can imagine yourself transmitting a brief surge of energy so that it gives him or her a boost for the day. I know healers who have mastered this practice to such an extent that they are able to perform an actual healing transaction in the brief moment of a handshake or hug. Similarly, you can learn to pass on undetected healing currents of energy through the ways you subtly touch others throughout the day.

Intimate Touch   In the realm of intimacy, the energetic view of life proposes that underneath sexual longing is the hope for an erotic union with the beloved, something that doesn't necessarily take place in our routine sexual conduct. When you shift to the practice of achieving highly resonant interactions with one another, you find out that it is possible for a sacred union of intimate partners to take place outside of traditional sexual practices, and this may occur in the bedroom or in public—for example, across the table in a restaurant. Autokinetics naturally brings you into new ways of exchanging energy with intimate others and leads you to reinvent your sex life by learning a variety of ways of achieving an energized union.

When your intimate partner joins you in the practice of Autokinetics, a whole new world of experience is opened for both of you. You can sit together and go through all of the three steps of the technique, in a way that synchronizes your movements. Follow the calling of your own body's desire to touch your partner, doing so in a way that makes way for a natural rhythm and movement to take over both of you. Be moved by the ways you can rock, sway, shake, vibrate, and touch together.

Undoubtably, one of the most incredible outcomes of Autokinetics is that it can supercharge your sex life. I often have heard couples say that they were completely surprised to discover how their energy breaks awakened new energy and desire for sexual expression. One couple from Fort Lauderdale, who had been married for nearly thirty years, used Autokinetics as a form of sexual play. They allowed their motions to flow spontaneously, falling into a kind of rhythmic trance that opened an intense experience of sexuality. As they moved together with more passion and desire, their bodies began to rock and sway until a powerful vibration moved through both of them at the same time. They actually felt that they were thrown into another reality, a place of complete bliss and ecstasy.

Many couples find this energetic sexual territory when they passionately engage in mutual Autokinetics. To their even greater surprise, they are sometimes able to reach a climax without actual physical intercourse. Instead, the power of mutually vibrating bodies moves each of them to have what I call a whole-body climax, an experience of becoming pure motion and vibration, truly a new frontier that warrants further exploration. These vibrational encounters—which some couples say are more satisfying than traditional forms of physical sexuality—may point us toward both safer and more pleasurable forms for the intimate exchange of energy, love, and passion.

I can assure you that when you enter the highest frequencies and vibrations with one another, a sensuality even more intense than conventional sexuality awaits you. There are spontaneous movements that can grab both of you, dissolve any sense of separateness, and bring you into a sacred union beyond what you had ever imagined possible.

Discovering the Ancient Mysteries of Life

The practice of Autokinetics prepares you for and opens you to the truths of the world's oldest spiritual traditions. In the natural movements of the universal life force you can be lifted into the highest realms of human experience. This is most likely to take place when you think less of your own immediate concerns and enter into a more intimate relationship with the whole of life. By becoming more empty of self and allowing the life force to surge through, you experience oneness with the universe.

When I first received a full transmission of the universal life force from Ikuko Osumi, Sensei, I began to feel as though my breath was inseparable from the breathing of all of life. With each breath, I experienced the whole universe breathe. In my practice of Autokinetics I have also felt my mind and body join with this universal breath.

Dr. Valerie Hunt of UCLA found that the highest vibrations we are capable of making bring us into the highest forms of mystical experience. She recorded the "mind field" frequency patterns of mystics who entered these realms and found it to be around 200 kilohertz, which was as high as the scientific measuring instruments in her laboratory could record. Compare this frequency with that of normal, grounded consciousness, less than 250 hertz, and that of psychic activity, somewhere above 400 hertz. What we find is that the highest mystical realms are associated with frequencies that are over 1,000 times greater than those associated with other states of consciousness. At the highest frequencies, people have a sense of luminosity, the "white light" that is referred to in near-death experiences and mystical episodes.

I believe that the highest frequencies Dr. Hunt describes are associated with the most energizing, revitalizing, and life-altering experiences we are capable of having. Here the deepest wisdom possible for anyone to encounter is brought directly into your being. You learn that the surest way to have energy, vitality, and happiness is to live considerately, kindly, and lovingly. As you give generously to others, the life force is brought into you. As you are kind to others, your life force is warmed and invigorated. And as you love in the highest way, the universal life force moves you to the supreme realms of mystical realization and attunement. In the heart of Autokinetics, the deepest pulse of life moves us to give and receive love.

Consequently, I agree with Dr. Robert Fulford that it is appropriate to see the whole universal life force as analagous to that which religions refer to as God, the divine, or the supreme being. This is what holds our life and is capable of healing and inspiring it. In this view, good is always associated with the unimpeded natural flow of life, whereas evil represents a blocking of this flow.

I have taught the movements of Autokinetics at the New York Open Center in New York City. There I had the opportunity to work with a young photographer who had spent nearly ten years living with a revered spiritual leader in India. When this photographer fell into the natural movements, he immediately entered a spiritual state of awareness and exclaimed that he was seeing the sacred light of the "divine mother." The natural movements brought him a profound spiritual experience that deeply touched his life.

In a ceremony of Autokinetic movement that I conducted several years ago in the San Francisco area, an internationally renowned concert pianist had a similar experience. The movements carried him into a powerful mystical experience that could be felt by all the people who witnessed it. His deep state opened his heart to the unimpeded flow of the life force.

I have seen insurance agents, interior decorators, schoolteachers, nurses, doctors, engineers, waitresses, clerks, painters, poets, carpenters, and computer programmers, to mention a few, have profound spiritual experiences that were initiated by simply allowing their bodies to be moved by the energy of life. As I have seen time and time again, no matter what spiritual tradition you belong to, or even if you do not actively adopt any particular tradition, the natural movements of Autokinetics can carry you into a sacred experience that may completely alter your life.

Energized Prayer

One of the surest ways to enter into the highest vibratory realms is through prayer. Alfred, Lord Tennyson, once wrote, "More things are wrought by prayer than this world dreams of." The pioneering work of Dr. Larry Dossey demonstrates that prayer is a powerfully effective medicine. Speaking about numerous research studies that show positive outcomes associated with praying, Dossey concludes, "If the technique studied [prayer] had been a new drug or a surgical procedure . . . it would almost certainly have been heralded as some kind of 'breakthrough.'"*

The key to the power of prayer in our lives is found in the way it moves us to positively resonate with the pulse of life itself, bringing us to the highest frequencies. Entering into an attitude of prayer is a way of tuning the mind and body to be more available to entering into the most powerful currents of the life force. Throughout the world, when people pray deeply and sincerely, they often rock back and forth. I have personally witnessed this spontaneous body movement in sacred services throughout the world, from the African-American Baptist church to the Bushmen's healing ceremony to the prayers given in an Orthodox Jewish synagogue.

The contemporary American healer Agnes Sanford, whose successes are well documented, always encouraged people to enter into energy healing with prayer. For believers, she would suggest saying something like, "Heavenly Father, please increase in me your life-giving power." For those who did not feel comfortable with those words, she would advise saying, "Whoever you are, whatever you are, come into me now." Such an act of prayer moves us to be less filled with ourselves and more filled with the larger field of life. The same spirit applies to the practice of Autokinetics. The vibrations and energy waves will come without prayer, but adding prayer gives you the supercharge. If you enter into it with an attitude and voice of handing yourself over to the *whole of life*, your practice will become more naturally empowered.

Although all ways of praying have been shown to work, I believe it is always good to ask that "Thy will be done" or, to say it differently,

---

*Larry Dossey, *Recovering the Soul: A Scientific and Spiritual Search*. New York: Bantam, 1989.

"May the whole of life take over." This final request moves us more deeply into a sacred relationship with life and attunes us to the most energizing and healing vibrations it offers.

As you move with the natural rhythms of life, you will find that your life becomes a spirited journey to quench your deepest thirst. By learning to move naturally with the pulse of life itself, you are returning to one of life's oldest truths. You discover, like Dorothy in *The Wizard of Oz,* that no matter how far you roam, if you keep moving you will find your way home. When you truly come home, you find a perfectly designed life awaiting you, one that is filled with kindness, grace, ecstatic joy, and blissful realization of your fondest hopes, desires, and dreams. Come home to the natural movements that are ready to energize and revitalize your life. There you can be reborn every day, bringing new energy and vitality to your personal journey. In the poetic words of Stanley Kunitz:

> *I can scarcely wait till tomorrow*
> *when a new life begins for me,*
> *as it does each day,*
> *as it does each day.*

CHAPTER FOUR

The Twelve Questions Most Often Asked

■_____

As I speak to audiences throughout the world about the way Autokinetics can powerfully charge their lives, I find that twelve questions are asked most often:

1. What is the most important thing I should remember when I take an energy break?

Always remember that you are heading toward the experience of having your body move with as little effort as possible on your part. This movement can be small or large, simple or complex, internal or external. When it feels automatic, it brings about a sense of calm, peace, and relaxation, and an absorbed state of mind. Again, the energy break brings a true recess into your life. When you were a kid, you were given a recess at school and allowed to play freely. As an adult, almost every second of your time is accounted for, and even when you get a break from work you use the time to get something done. When you exercise or relax, it's probably done in a purposeful way. Rarely, if ever, do you give your body a chance to be free and allow it to move in its own way. By bringing more moments of true recess into your life, your body is not only able to relax; it is able to tune itself and help move you into a more energized state of being.

2. Are there any foods that would give me more energy?

What is most important about what you eat is the amount of energy
your body has in order to metabolize it. If you have little life force, you
won't be able to get much value out of the best foods in the world,
whereas if you are filled with the life force you will be able to maximize the nutritional value of any food. To understand the unique
relationship you have with food, one thing you can do is to keep track
of what happens to you when you eat certain foods. Carry a notebook,
write down what you eat, and keep notes on how you feel afterward.
This self-study can reveal foods and combinations of foods that are a
problem for you. For example, some foods are not a problem when
eaten alone, but they may drain you if they are eaten together with certain other foods. Find which foods make you more energized and
which ones leave you with a headache, fatigue, or disorientation. I
personally find that spinach is the most powerful energy food and will
help most people build up their life force. Popeye the sailor obviously
knew what practitioners of Chinese medicine have always known
about spinach as a source of energy and vitality.

3. Can the energy break help keep me young?

I have seen people look dramatically younger after they practiced
Autokinetics for a year or two. In Japan, the patients of Ikuko Osumi,
Sensei, refer to this kind of energizing practice as a "fountain of
youth." I have met people who, after practicing this technique every
day for more than ten years, looked ten to twenty years younger than
they actually were. It is the life force that gives you the essence of
youth—that is, the vitality and glow of being vibrantly alive. The
secret of maintaining youth has little to do with health tonics, skin
conditioners, enzyme treatments, or formulas. This secret can't be

purchased at a spa or health food store. It is the universal life force, and it it is free and available everywhere on earth.

4. Do I have to sit to take an energy break?

Listen to the calling of your own body. If you feel drawn to stand or move about, then do so. I have found that most of the time we are more likely to fall into the natural movements while sitting and rocking. But, again, listen to your teacher—the natural movements of your own body.

5. Can music help me do the energy break?

Over the years I have experimented with various kinds of music, rhythms, and sounds that will facilitate this practice. Not all music helps. If music is too melodic or draws you into familiar ways of expressing yourself, then it may not help you fall into the natural movements required for this orientation. What you need is a musical and rhythmic background that pulses in a manner that helps bring you into resonance with the life force.

6. Will the energy break improve my sex life?

It is very common for Autokinetics to bring new energy into your sex life. Sexuality is one expression of the life force, with its vibratory states, rhythmic movements, and waves of energy. Ancient traditions have long known about the relationship of sexuality to the life force and have prescribed a wide variety of ways to use one to affect the other. It's a great idea to encourage your intimate partner to do Autokinetics with you. This will open new ways of moving the life force into your sex life and will bring more delight, pleasure, and eros into your practice.

7. I'm a senior citizen and want to know whether I'm too old to take an energy break with Autokinetics.

Autokinetics is perfect for senior citizens. Because it invites only those movements that are natural and effortless, there is no concern with straining or hurting yourself. It will bring new vitality and energy into your daily life, as well as open you to creative ideas for projects that will help you initiate more inspiring activity.

Throughout Asia, daily work with life energy is common for people of all ages. There you find that older people who have a daily practice of bringing the life force into the body appear to get younger rather than older with age. Their faces glow with brightness, and they are sometimes able to outperform adults who are twenty years younger.

As you move into the most advanced age group, Autokinetics will continue to bring benefits to your life. It can improve your digestion and bladder control, strengthen your muscles and bones, improve your sleeping patterns, relieve itching skin (one of the most common problems of old age), and bring about a daily sense of being restored and revitalized.

I believe that Autokinetics offers unlimited benefits to senior citizens, who often fight a daily battle with fatigue and are looking for a source of energy that can revitalize their lives. I'm convinced that all retirement communities and all retired people should know about this simple and safe practice and bring it into their everyday life.

8. I am a spiritual person who believes in the power of prayer. How can this be integrated with Autokinetics?

I encourage people to practice what I call "energized praying." This involves saying your prayer while you are in an energized state. When your body moves with the pulse of the life force, ask to be lifted into the highest frequencies that bring forth the spiritual resonances. As your body moves into these realms of vibratory experience, say your prayer with the belief that it is empowered and centered in the heart of spirituality.

9. I am not able to move parts of my body because of illness [or injury]. How should I do an energy break?

Since there is no right or wrong movement, do not worry about what part of your body moves and what doesn't move. Allow the natural rhythms to play themselves on you in their own way. You may move only your fingers or toes, or you may only feel a vibration within your body. You may also explore visualizing or feeling imaginary movements of injured parts of your body. This will bring energy to them and contribute to your whole well-being.

10. When did human beings first recognize the healing power of the life force?

Although I assume that the world's oldest cultures have always healed themselves with the life force, there is no written account of the life force until around 2000 B.C. That is when the world's first medical document was written, *The Yellow Emperor's Book of Internal Medicine*, which presents the concept of a body energy called *chi* or *qi*. In this Chinese text we find these words: "If your energy is strong, no illness can befall you," and "If illness strikes, it is because your energy is weak."

Another ancient Chinese belief is that qi is made up of two complementary aspects: yin and yang. When these two aspects or forces are balanced, a state of health naturally develops. However, when they are unbalanced, the stage is set for disease. The ancient Chinese learned to direct as well as balance the life energy as a means of preventing disease and premature aging.

Throughout the world, we find historical evidence of an awareness of the life force. Some scholars speculate that the spiritual masters of India learned to circulate the energy in their bodies and with that of another person as long ago as 5000 B.C. Ancient Egypt also had knowledge of the healing energy that could come about through a laying on of hands. Kabbalah, the ancient Jewish mystical tradition, refers to this energy as the astral light. The art of working with the life force may be said to be as old as human culture.

11. Are there more advanced teachings and suggestions that are helpful as I become more experienced with Autokinetics?

There are more things to be learned that I haven't talked about in this book, because they wouldn't make sense unless you were first accustomed to the energizing practice. That information will be made available in a forthcoming work.

12. Will the energy break help me achieve success in my life?

Without a doubt, energy is the most powerful way to help you achieve the success you desire. Not only does it fill you with the vitality neeeded to actualize your potential; it brings personal guidance, confidence, and a deep trust in the natural processes of life. Energizing your life is the first step toward realizing the life you most desire. It helps you find the right goals for yourself—those that are most natural—and it brings you into the wisdom of life itself. Here you find the path that has heart and the journey that brings back the mystery and wonder we once felt as children. By bringing you back to your true origins, it helps you find the surest way to your future dreams and victories.

CHAPTER FIVE

Life Energy in Ancient and Modern Traditions

Throughout the world, different cultures have found their own unique way to the life force. Whether or not there is a pounding drum, a shaking rattle, an ecstatic dance, a solemn prayer, or a meditative posture, underneath all traditions is the steady pulse of a body that moves in sync with the energy of life. I will present some of the different ways that life energy is moved into the human body, beginning with more subtle forms of energy work and then moving on to forms that involve more ecstatic processes, such as a shaking body or a frenzied ceremonial dance. I will look at a variety of traditions, old and new, from all over the world, emphasizing those I have experienced firsthand.

The Physician's Healing Touch

The history of Western medical science is rooted in the gentle and subtle practice of passing healing energy through touch. In ancient Greece there was a cult surrounding the physician Aesculapius, who was called the "divine physician" or "gentle healer." His followers, including Hippocrates, practiced a laying on of hands that they believed transferred a healing power to their patients. The Hippocratic oath, still quoted by today's physicians, begins with an acknowledgment to this tradition: "I swear by Apollo the physician, by Aesculapius . . . to keep according to my ability and my judgment the following oath . . ." The physician and renowned author Lewis Thomas was well aware of this ancient contribution of touch to medicine. As he stated, "Touching is medicine's oldest secret, never acknowledged as the central, essential skill and always obscured by the dancing and the chanting—but always busily there, the laying on of hands."*

Among nurses, "therapeutic touch" has received widespread acceptance in contemporary times. Developed by Dolores Krieger, a professor of nursing at New York University, this orientation teaches you to work with the subtle currents of the life force. More than 30,000 nurses in the United States and Canada now use this energy healing in hospitals and clinics. Krieger was responsible for an often quoted research study, which found that "when ill people are treated by the laying on of hands, a significant change occurs in the hemoglobin component of their red blood cells."† This kind of research is continuing throughout the medical community, particularly at facilities like the Touch Research Institute, the world's first scientific facility devoted to the study of touch, at the University of Miami School of Medicine.

*Lewis Thomas, *The Lives of a Cell*. New York: Viking, 1974.

†See Dolores Krieger, "The Relationship of Touch, with Intent to Help or Heal, to Subjects' In-vivo Hemoglobin Values: A Study in Personalized Interactions," Proceedings, American Nurses Association Ninth Nursing Research Conference, San Antonio, Texas, March 21–23, 1973, pp. 39–58, and Daniel Benor, *Healing Research: Holistic Energy Medicine and Spiritual Healing*, Volume 1. London: Helix Editions, 1993.

The Christian Tradition of Touch

The Christian tradition gave rise to what was called the "royal touch." At one time in English history, healing through touch was considered a sign that a person had the right to occupy the throne. Since monarchs were thought to be divinely chosen, it was believed that they had the gift of healing. In 1732, the surgeon William Beckett conducted an official investigation of the royal touch and declared that it was effective. He hypothesized that being near the king aroused such excitement that the sick person's blood flow increased, causing a healing to take place.

Many Christian healing services today favor a more settled, relaxed form of laying on of the hands that does not encourage wild ecstatic body movements. But some churches may allow a mild form of body movement such as raising the arms and waving the hands; still others may permit jumping up and down, though they frown upon dancing. The movements that are accepted are those that the religious leaders are comfortable with. There is no right or wrong way of moving with the life force, and people should move into it in a way that is most natural for them, whether it be in the frenzied dancing of an ecstatic religious service or rock concert or a calmer, and gentler form.

A wonderful introduction to the Christian practice of laying on hands is found in Malcolm Miner's book *Your Touch Can Heal: A Guide to Healing Touch and How to Use It.* The author, a former college chaplain, priest, and president of the International Order of Saint Luke the Physician, became involved in healing touch by accident as his ministry called on him to be with the sick. There he found that people could be healed if he touched them as he prayed. He gives the same advice that is taught by elders throughout the world: no matter what your worldview happens to be, the strongest work takes place when you believe that the energy coming through you is from the *highest good.*

Chinese Energy Medicine

In China and throughout Asia there are ancient traditions of working with the life force that are sometimes called "subtle energy" practices. They usually involve one person's passing energized hands over another person's body while transmitting *qi*, that is, subtle currents of the life force. "External qi healing" (*wai qi zhi liao*) is a common therapy in Chinese hospitals. The healer projects qi, the vital life force, through his or her own body in order to affect the energy field of the patient. Rooted in the ancient practice of *qi gong*, which literally means "working with life energy," this method has been studied scientifically in the Shanghai College of Traditional Chinese Medicine, where laboratory animals with cancer were given qi and found to survive longer than those who did not receive it. Chinese researchers have even introduced the notion of a qi gong EEG. This pattern of electrical activity in the brain takes place both in the person transmitting the energy and in the person receiving it.

There are between 2,000 and 4,000 different styles of qi gong in China. These approaches to working with the life force teach body movements that can be done while lying, sitting, or standing. The Shanghai Qi Gong Research Institute was the first institution devoted to the scientific study of qi gong. There and in other Chinese research settings, qi gong has been found to improve health, energy, stamina, and the quality of daily work. Scientific research in China validates that moving the life force in your body helps relieve stress, eliminate jet lag, improve sports performance, charge the immune system, relieve acute and chronic pain, speed recovery from injuries, and increase the effectiveness of Western medicines. It has been found to reduce the healing time after surgery by 50 percent and has been found effective in healing tuberculosis, gastric and duodenal ulcers, liver disease, nearsightedness, substance abuse, obesity, asthma, and allergies. It also provides benefits to people suffering from neuromuscular difficulties such as poststroke syndrome, paralysis from spinal cord injuries, multiple sclerosis, Parkinson's disease, cerebral palsy, and aphasia.

There are also more than thirty research studies in China claiming that moving the life force in the body through qi gong has reversed the aging process. The effects of qi on the body include a reduced incidence of stroke, improved EKG (heart) readings, and lower levels of blood sugar in diabetics. There are estimated to be more than 1 million cancer patients in China who practice qi gong on a daily basis, with numerous reports of remissions. Qi gong has also been found to reduce or completely eliminate the side effects of chemotherapy.

Chinese master teachers of qi will sometimes challenge a student to hit them as hard as possible, but the student who tries is repelled away from the teacher's body, sometimes falling to the ground. The masters claim that they are able to do this by sending out waves of qi that stop anyone from touching them. One of my students, William Sutherland, has experienced this firsthand and reports that it is like running into a force field that takes all the energy out of your muscles.

The central belief behind qi gong is that besides our nervous and circulatory systems, we also have energy pathways—these are called meridians—distributed throughout the body. Two French medical doctors, Jean-Claude Darras and Pierre de Vernejoul, have conducted experiments at the nuclear medicine section of the Necker Hospital in Paris that they believe confirm the existence of these energy channels. They injected a solution of isotopes into different points on a subject's body, identified by the Chinese as energy spots—these are called acupoints—and then traced them with gamma-camera imaging. They found that the isotopes clearly moved along the classical Chinese energy pathways.

In addition to qi gong, there are numerous other Eastern orientations to energy work. These include acupressure, *shiatsu, chi nei tsang, anma, hoshino, jin shin jyutsu, ayurveda,* and *t'ai chi chuan,* as well as many schools of kundalini yoga, aikido, and karate. Scholars speculate that there were vibratory energy practitioners in China as long as 10,000 years ago.

The Kundalini of India

In India there is great familiarity with the universal life force and how it may bring waves of energy into your body, causing major changes in your whole being. This is typically called a "kundalini awakening." A yoga may first experience the energy at the base of the spine, as if it were a coiled spring or snake waiting to be awakened. In fact, the Sanskrit word *kundalini* actually means "coiled up," and the term is used to refer to the coiled energy that lives within us, waiting to be aroused and brought into every aspect of our life. Once activated, the energy may crawl slowly up the spine or flood the body like a geyser. The energy may circulate inside the body or flow out of the crown of your head. When this happens, the body vibrates or feels electrically charged, and a wide array of sensory experiences are possible, usually involving sensations of heat, light, and sound.

The great spiritual traditions of India have devised anatomies and physiologies of the energized body, referring to the main energy stations as *cakras* (often transliterated as *chakras*). Usually depicted as lotus flowers with varying numbers of petals, they represent different vortices of energy that are arrayed along the body's axis. The tantra yoga theory of kundalini goes on to propose several ducts or passageways, called *nadi,* along which the charged kundalini travels. Various yoga traditions prescribe different ways of activating this energy and moving it through the body as a spiritual practice. These include the use of sound, spontaneous hand gestures and body movements, and specialized meditative postures. It is generally believed that as a result of a full, mature awakening, this energy will move upward from the bottom of the spine, through each chakra, and finally out of the body and into the center of the universal life force itself, producing an experience of enlightenment. People who are fully initiated into this deepest communion with life are said to be naturally connected to a universal wisdom that helps them teach and help others.

Shaking the Energized Body Throughout the world I have found many diverse cultures that have their own unique way of working with the universal life force. In Nova Scotia, the blind Micmac medicine man, Dave Gehue, naturally feels in his body, the force of life which causes him to shake and touch others with his healing touch. His teacher, the late Cree elder Albert Lightning, was also a "shaker" and would find his body seized with the life force. Gehue believes that the strongest medicine people always shake with the life force. As he said to me, "No shake, no shaman."

A body that shakes and vibrates with the life force is perhaps the truest sign of someone entering the ecstatic state of shamanism, the oldest religious practice on earth. The word *shaman* is of Siberian origin, and scholars have proposed that it originally referred to the excited, shaking body of the shaman. This is sometimes forgotten in contemporary understanding and expressions of shamanism, where the primary emphasis is upon using a technique of guided imagery to direct an inner fantasy journey to another realm. For the shamans I have met around the world, having such a flight is only one of the experiences that are possible. What is most central to their practice, however, is having the energy or spirit of life enter their body, where it vibrates, ripples, and shakes them with its currents.

No matter what culture you visit in the world, the surest way to find its practice of working with the universal life force is to find some-one—a medicine person, shaman, healer, priest, or spiritual teacher—whose body moves and shakes when he or she is helping others.

Shaking Among the Ojibway Indians   Sometimes the shaking, en-ergized body of the healer is hidden from the view of others. For example, among the Ojibway Indians in Canada and the north-central United States, one of the most powerful healing ceremonies is referred to as the "shaking tent." In this ceremony a medicine man enters a special tent made of sticks firmly dug into the ground and covered with hide or cloth, with bells hanging from the top, which is open to the sky. When the medicine man enters this tent, shakes his rattle, and sings his sacred song, the tent begins to move back and forth wildly, sometimes looking as though it might fly out of the ground. In this state of mind, the medicine man is available for spiritual consul-tation and healing encounters with members of the community who have come for help.

What usually takes place in the shaking tent ceremony is that the medicine man's body is filled with the life force, resulting in an ener-gized body that moves the tent with almost superhuman strength. A description of what the medicine man typically does inside this tent was given by the anthropologist A. Irving Hallowell in 1942:

> *The conventional position which the conjurer is supposed to as-sume in the lodge is one of the commonly made sitting postures. The*

knees rest on the ground and the buttocks against the heels. It is the ordinary posture of a canoeman paddling in the bow; but in the conjuring lodge [shaking tent] the upper part of the body is bent forward until the head almost touches the ground . . . with his right hand the conjurer grasps one of the upright poles not far from the ground. As soon as he does so he "feels something strange," I was told, and the structure begins to vibrate.*

The Yuwipi Ceremony of the Lakota Indians   The shaking body of the medicine man is often hidden from view in Native Americans' ceremonies, perhaps because it is their belief that shaking is a sign of the movement of spirit rather than the movement of the healer's body, or because there is simply some shyness about displaying a frenzied ecstatic state. The Lakota Indians call one of their most sacred ceremonies *yuwipi*, which means "they bind him." Here the medicine man is wrapped in a star quilt, bound with rope, and laid on the floor in the dark. The singers and drummers call forth the spirits, while, unseen to the community, the medicine man's body is powerfully shaken, resulting in his being freed from the rope and able to shake rattles and move about in a fully energized way. Again, the shaking state of the medicine man's body is hidden and kept secret from noninitiates, for reasons that can only be hypothesized.

I cannot make the claim that all medicine men who practice the shaking tent, yuwipi, or other spirit-summoning ceremonies do so through a body energized by the life force. But I can say that all the healers who have shared their work with me have indicated this, and

---

*From A. Irving Hallowell, *The Role of Conjuring in Salteaux Society.* Philadelphia: University of Pennsylvania Press, 1942, p. 42.

that my own experience of these ceremonies also indicates it. Even when these medicine people are unwilling to believe that the phenomena associated with their work are caused by an energized body, they will still admit that the body is shaking and moving when the spirits are present.

Shaking in the Church   But you don't have to go to a Native American reservation to see the life force move a human body. Go to any spirit-filled African-American church on a Sunday morning, and you will see bodies vibrating, dancing, trembling, and shaking in the same way that is seen in the healing ceremonies of Africa. I have attended many of these church services and found their use of rhythm and music to have the same effect on their parishioners as on tribal members in the middle of an African village, where elephant-hide drums are played and the shrieking sounds of *sangomas,* or medicine people, lead a community into a state of ecstatic energy.

The energized movement of bodies in the church historically extends beyond the African-American churches. The early Quakers were so named because of the energized trembling that they experienced in their religious services. A Quaker historian noted that their movements were so intense that "on one occasion the house itself seemed to be shaken."

The rise of Methodism in England was also filled with energized bodies, as John Wesley writes:

> *While I was earnestly inviting all men to enter into the Holiest by this new and living way, many of those that heard began to call upon God with strong cries and tears. . . . Others exceedingly trembled and quaked. Some were torn with a kind of convulsive motion*

in every part of their bodies so that . . . four or five persons could not hold them. *

Similarly, the Shakers of England came to America in 1780 partly because of the discomfort other people felt while watching the energized states that led them to publicly dance, shout, and shake. F. W. Evans, a nineteenth-century Shaker, wrote of their energized movement in 1859, in a compendium on the history and practice of their faith:

> *Sometimes, after sitting a while in silent meditation, they were seized with a mighty trembling . . . They were often exercised with great agitation of body and limbs, shaking, running, and walking the floor, with a variety of other operations and signs swiftly passing and repassing each other like clouds agitated with a mighty wind.*†

Indian Shakers   In a classic scholarly study entitled *Indian Shakers*, H. G. Barnett tells the history of a cult of Native American shakers in the Pacific Northwest. Their spiritual shaking began in 1881 when a forty-year-old Indian from Puget Sound named John Slocum fell sick and appeared to be dying. His wife, Mary Slocum, went into a fit of praying, trembling, and wild shaking. This started when she felt something hot flow over her body, making her body tremble. After she

---

*Cited in Robert Southey, *The Life of Wesley and the Rise and Progress of Methodism.* New York, 1847.

†Cited in F. W. Evans, *Shakers: Compendium of the Origin, History, Principles, Rules and Regulations, Government, and Doctrines of the United Society of Believers in Christ.* New York, 1859.

touched her husband, he was healed, and her shaking was immediately held to be a powerful medicine. She took no credit for what had taken place and insisted that what happened to her could happen to anyone. She then demonstrated how her shaking could be transmitted from one person to another. The *shake,* as a medicine, was found to have curative and revitalizing properties that brought about physical and mental relief.

These Indian Shakers, as they came to be known, still exist today. Sometimes they have visions when they are under the influence of an energized, shaking body, enabling them to find lost objects, see the future, and foretell deaths and sickness.

In their rituals, Indian Shakers fall into a dance that has similarities to the healing dance of the Kalahari Bushmen. The Indian Shakers move in and out of the dance until shaking comes upon someone. That person then places his or her fluttering hands on another person's body, in the same manner that you would see in the Bushmen's energized ceremony.

Throughout the world we find reports of people falling into dances and movements that stir up an ecstatic state and fill them with a new sense of life and vitality. This was true of the ghost-dancers at Wounded Knee—and of the early gnostics, whose sacred dance, according to Elaine Pagels's *The Gnostic Gospels,* was originally led by Jesus. Whether it be the whirling dervishes of Turkey, who spin around and around to enter the mystical realm, or the swaying movement of worshipers in a Jewish synagogue, there is a natural process, reported throughout human history, that involves falling into spontaneous movements, which opens a door to energized bodies and ecstatic states of consciousness.

The Energy Dance of the Bushmen

I once dreamed of going to the Kalahari Desert and dancing with the Bushmen, the oldest living people of Africa. Within several years my dream was realized, and I found myself living among a group of Bushmen in an isolated part of the Kalahari Desert near the southern border of Khutse National Park in Botswana. There I experienced their healing dance, fell into its trance, and felt their healing energy move throughout my body. I talked with their elders and healers and learned both from their words and from their healing hands how it is possible to bring the vital life force directly into your own body.

For the Bushmen the name of this spiritual energy is *num,* and they believe it to be a medicine that is capable of healing us and giving us vitality. They often dance nightlong ceremonies to bring forth this *num* and to circulate it into the body of everyone who is present. It is as vital to their life as the air they breathe and the food that they eat. When you live among the Bushmen, you quickly see that although we are living with breath and food, we have lost touch with the revitalizing nourishment that is provided from a steady diet of the universal life force.

I believe that the Bushmen's healing dance is the purest form of healing to be found anywhere in the world. Even many of Africa's great healers—including Credo Mutwa, one of the spiritual leaders of the traditional Zulu people—believe that the energy coming from the Bushmen's healing dance is the strongest medicine in Africa and possibly on earth. Anthropologists have intensively filmed, studied, and written about these extraordinary rituals, where men and women enter deep trancelike states and lay their fluttering hands on everyone in the community as a means of energizing one another. The South African writer Sir Laurens van der Post described his impression of their dance in this way:

[They] surrendered to it without reservation, shame or consciousness of any kind . . . I felt as if the whole of the Universe had come to a point at that moment. Never had I heard human voices go so far back in time, so deeply down into the pit of being. This I thought was the cry of longing, anguish, and desire of the first man on earth. The music and the voices reached a depth of intensity in the human body which I would have not thought possible. . . . I can only say that I myself have never felt more dedicated and nearer God than at that moment and stood there almost in tears as one with revelation in a temple.*

One of the things that makes the Bushmen unique is that they do not limit their healing practice to a few special initiates, but make it avilable to anyone who wants to experience it. They do not hesitate to talk about their healing practice, and they invite you to come to their dance and try it for yourself. They are completely free with their spirituality and their ancient wisdom, while at the same time they are aware that they are speaking about something that is practically impossible to describe unless you have experienced it firsthand.

Num Is Everywhere When I first met the Bushmen, I was told that *num,* the sacred energy of life, is everywhere. It is in the earth, in the air around us, in the fire that blazes in the center of their healing dance, in the spirited rhythms and songs of passionate and soulful music, and in the motion of ecstatic dance. When we feel the initial stirring of this energy inside the body, it is like a tingling sensation. It may be a rippling wave or two of excitement, or it may express itself

---

*Laurens van der Post, "The Creative Pattern in Primitive Africa," Eranus Lectures. Dallas, Texas, Spring, 1957, pp. 16–17.

as an intermittent inner buzzing that is related to our anticipation and belief that something important is about to happen. Each of us has felt this inner stirring of energy, whether before a first date or a first kiss, or at the beginning of a championship game, during the opening music of a long-awaited concert, at the raising of the curtain to reveal the first scene of a blockbuster Broadway play, or at the first cry of a newborn baby. This energy of excitement is the energy of life, something that flows through us when we are perfectly tuned to a soul-stirring event that is taking place right in front of us.

What a Bushman does when he or she feels this inner stirring is to step into it and allow it to escalate so that the energy grows in intensity and strength. As the *num,* or life force, is heated up and moves toward the boiling point, the dancing Bushmen approach a point where they, too, become nervous and concerned about whether they want to go all the way and let this energy completely take over. When they surrender to it, they feel a silencing of the psychological self and they lose themselves completely to the energy. They refer to this full crossing over into the *num* as a death experience—a passing over into a state where the energy of life—rather than the voice of control and understanding articulated by their inner self—takes over the mind and body.

Bushman Healing   When these Bushmen go all the way into this energy, they become pure instruments of healing. The whole body becomes filled with *num,* and they are able to walk through a gathering of people and send the energy into everyone. When they are doing this, what you see is an energetic form of laying their hands on the bodies of others. Hands, limbs, and the whole body vibrate in a rhythm that resonates with seven to eight beats per second. Sometimes healers wrap their arms and legs around the person they are working with or even lie down across the other person's body, either crosswise or lengthwise, while the healer's whole body shakes, helping the other person enter into this vibrational state. During this movement, the *num* songs are sung with a pulse that is also moving between seven to eight beats per second.* In this music, which is filled with improvisational complexity, energy is generated and sent into the air, providing still another source of transmission of the universal life force.

In the excited state of a body filled with *num*, the Bushmen are said to be in *kia*, an enhanced state of consciousness that is required for passing on the healing energy. In this state, the whole range of spiritual and transcendent experience is available to the recipient. Visionary journeys into the spirit world, extraordinary psychic events, handling and walking on fire, intuitive diagnosis, seeing inside the bodies of others, viewing events far away from their camp, immersion into spiritual luminosity, and healing others may all take place. Being filled with *num*, the universal life force, opens the doors to a powerfully vibrant spiritual life where every known spiritual experience is available.

Those who allow their *num* to boil may enter deep spiritual territory. To cross into this place requires moving past the fear of death. Bushmen sometimes emphasize that this entry requires experiencing what they consider a real death, rather than what we might be tempted to regard as a symbolic one. This ordeal is the final "letting go" before the soul is free to roam the spiritual universe. No longer do they bind the soul to the limitations of mind and body. It becomes instantaneously connected to all places in the spiritual universe. Through

---

*First observed by N. England, *Music Among the Zu/Wasi of South Western Africa and Botswana*. Ph.D. dissertation, Harvard University, Cambridge, Mass., 1968.

boiling energy they enter the realm of the mystic and of the spiritual visionaries who find their way into the eyes and ears of the divine.

However, one does not have to go all the way into this energy to benefit from it. Not everyone at a Bushman healing ceremony goes into *kia*. Some simply tune themselves to receive the energy as a means of revitalizing the body and their general well-being. Others enter into *kia* but don't escalate it into the state where they are naturally moved to energize and heal others. Not all Bushmen make a complete surrender to it, and no matter how many times you have done it, you start from scratch at each new ceremonial gathering. Most Bushmen have the experience of fully entering this energy state at least once in their lives, but not all choose to do so on a regular basis. Those who do so are regarded as the healers of the community.

These masters of *num*, called *num kausi*, are said to possess *num* in the base of the spine and the pit of the stomach. When they activate or awaken it, their bodies sweat profusely as the *num* begins to boil. This boiling turns the *num* into a vapor that rises up the spine and enters the base of the skull, bringing forth the experience of *kia*. As a Bushman healer put it, "The *num* makes me boil and tremble and shakes out my thoughts so that there is only the *num* inside me. It moves my body and hands to touch others and brings the *num* into them."

The healing work of the Bushmen also draws upon the spontaneous use of incredible sounds—sometimes crying, shrieking, wailing, whistling, gasping, grunting, screaming, and almost ear-shattering noises. These sounds carry the life force, and their vibrations are as healing as the laying on of hands. As the energized healer applies his or her hands to another person's body, these sounds may be shouted out or actually voiced into the other person's body.

Anyone who is present at one of these ceremonies will automatically become tuned by the pulse of its energy and will receive its revitalizing current. Even the little children and babies of the community are touched and moved by the natural expression of this energy. The Bushmen readily accept that this energy is required for health and well-being. Furthermore, the *num* songs are sung throughout the day, bathing everyday activities in vitalizing energy.

The Bushmen believe that what is important to learn about this energy work cannot be taught in a classroom but is born out of fresh experience. With this in mind, it is not surprising that they are not much concerned with preserving their past knowledge, and they do not place any major emphasis on systematically teaching it to their children. The implication for us is that the force of life itself will teach you how to revitalize and heal yourself.

Perhaps more than any people on our planet, the Bushmen have a day-to-day awareness of and relationship to the universal life force that provide us with an example of what it would be like to live a fully charged life. Not only are the healing dances available each week and energizing songs sung throughout the day; the Bushmen may jump on any occasion that presents itself with a spark of energy. For instance, if a couple or group were sitting around holding a conversation or telling a joke, one person might suddenly feel the onset of an inner tingling of energy. If he or she gives in to this energy and allows it to escalate into a strong current, all the others immediately stop what they are doing and physically gather close to one another so that the recently awakened energy may be moved into each person's body. They may even start singing a *num* song and falling into the healing dance. As soon as the energy has subsided, they immediately go back to what they were doing, finishing their conversation or completing the joke that someone was in the middle of sharing. In this way, energy and healing work are beautifully interwoven into the fabric of everyday life. There are no special places or specially anointed people to regulate and control the spiritual and healing aspect of life. It is free and available to everyone.

The Bushman's Way of Moving Life Energy　When I was with the Bushmen, they taught me their way of moving the universal life force into the body. This energy work begins by catching a little energy ripple or vibration. When you go fishing, you typically throw out your line with some bait attached to the hook. You then sit and wait until you feel a little nibble on that hook. When you feel that momentary movement, you try to catch the fish and reel it in. Similarly, in this energy work you bait yourself to catch some universal life force. You do those things that are most likely to send a momentary ripple or tingle of energy through your body. The Bushmen use rhythm, spirited music, soulful dancing, playful teasing, flirtation, spicy humor, and spontaneous, improvised sounds and movements to jump-start themselves. These activities are like bait that helps you catch an energy wave. When this playful activity sends a ripple of energy your way, you try to bring it into your body so that it connects you with the never-ending pulse of the universal life energy. In other words, you try to catch this energy so that it can enter you. Perhaps it is more accurate to say that you set up a situation where you are likely to be caught by the energy of life. You actually feel as if you are caught by its rippling currents because when it catches you, your movements and actions become automatic, spontaneous, and effortless.

　　I remember the first time I danced with the Bushmen. Underneath a starry sky in the Kalahari, amidst the polyrhythms of singing and rattling cocoons wrapped around their ankles, I felt the energy of the dance literally jump into my hips. Without effort my legs and body were moved, and the dance energized my body. As I went deeper into its flow, I went into that state of mind that transcends our use of language and had the kind of magical awareness that enables you to understand what people are communicating, whether or not you consciously know their language or whether they even speak a single word. There I was able to feel the life force vibrate itself through my whole body and to experience firsthand how my whole being could be used as an intermediary or midwife for the passage of this current into the bodies of other people.

Nothing is more ecstatic, invigorating, revitalizing, and blissful than powerful currents of life's energy filling every cell of your body and moving with it without any restriction or constraint. I have never stopped dancing with the energy the Bushmen introduced me to, and rarely does a week go by when I don't immerse myself in its strongest currents and deepest wells.

The Bushmen taught me that there are many kinds of experiences with the universal life force that are available to us in everyday life. These include pausing for a few seconds to get a quick charge, setting aside a time for a brief tune-up that reconnects you to life's revitalizing flow, to a full, lengthy immersion in its most powerful currents.

The Bushmen also taught me the importance of maintaining light-heartedness about this work. Before each ceremony they tease each other and even tell sexual jokes, always laughing and preserving the spirit of play and levity. After the ceremony has taken someone on a deep plunge into the energy, someone else may again tease or joke in order to provide a moment of comic relief. Frivolity is also interspersed thoroughout those times when people are on a rest cycle in the midst of ceremonial work. Humor and absurdity therefore serve as a way of lightening our spirit to enter into and out of our deep plunges into the ocean of life's energy.

The other lesson that the Bushmen can teach us involves how they often create a healing social group whose energy is encouraged to exceed that of any individual healer. This takes place when people's bodies tremble and shake in rhythm with one another. The combination of these equal-frequency vibrations brings on a greatly amplified movement of the life force. Whether they are praying together, singing together, or healing together, when the activity is coordinated so that the movements of each person are in sync with those of the others, a powerful group effect is created. Not only does this bring greater energy into the person being healed; it brings more healing energy to each group member.

Bushmen elders speak of the "awakening of *num*" as an "awakening of their hearts," because if their hearts weren't awakened, they wouldn't care enough to make any effort to heal others. The energy dance is held not only to heal and revitalize, but also to ignite their longing to have ecstatic experiences with one another. Anyone may call for a dance, and it may be held for no other reason than to have good old-fashioned fun and excitement. But once the dance begins and the energy begins to boil, everyone is joined together in the purpose of this energy: revitalizing the well-being of all who come to the gathering. Those who bring in the energy are there to pass it on to others.

Although anthropologists and field observers have tried to make generalizations about the healing practices of the Bushmen, I personally found that the Bushmen themselves neither value nor pay much attention to such conceptual generalizations. They value the improvisational, experimental nature of their healing energy work. I don't think there can be a true generalization about healing by the Bushmen except to say that it originates in the universal life force and is orchestrated by that force. The Bushmen move as the *num* calls them to move. They fall into natural attunement with the energy of life, allow it to be stirred, and hand over their bodies and minds to be used for the soulful and spirited expression of life. The life of the Bushmen exemplifies the ease with which we, too, may fall into these movements and become revitalized by them.

The Bushmen and other indigenous people from all around the world have something to teach us that is of vital importance. They can show us how to live with more than bread, breath, and water. They point us toward the source of life itself, the never-ending flow of energy that is capable of revitalizing every part of the body, mind, and soul.

One night under a full moon in the Kalahari Desert, Sir Laurens van der Post asked a Bushman why they danced throughout the night. His Bushman friend gave him a bewildered look and said: "From now on the moon will begin to fade away and unless we show the moon how much our hearts love the light of the moon it will fade utterly away and not come back but die."* This image provides an important teaching: In our natural state of attunement our hearts open to the light of life. In the heart of life we become the moon and bring light to one another. As the Bushmen say, "You must henceforth be the moon. You must shine at night. By your shining you shall light the darkness for men until the sun rises again to light up all things."

The Aborigines' Dreamtime Energy

If you travel along the Tropic of Capricorn, the latitude that crosses through the Bushmen's home in the Kalahari Desert, you will eventually find yourself walking straight into the home of the world's

---

*Laurens van der Post, "The Creative Pattern in Primitive Africa," Eranus Lectures, Dallas, Texas, Spring, 1957, p. 40.

other oldest culture, the Aborigines of Australia. They, too, have long been familiar with how to gain access to the universal life force. In their most secret ceremonies they allow their bodies to vibrate and resonate with the pulse of what they believe is the "Dreamtime."

The Aborigines believe that nature has a mind that is capable of dreaming. They enter this dreaming by tuning themselves to be in perfect resonance with their natural surroundings. When they pulse with nature in the right way, they become inseparable from nature, and it then becomes natural to dream with nature. In this expanded mind, they have access to information about things that are outside of the boundaries of their sensory processes. In our culture, such awareness is often called a psychic talent, and is believed to be the special gift of a chosen few. Among Aborigines, it is regarded as being as natural as seeing a kangaroo hop across the Australian landscape. They know that our mind may be expanded into the Mind of Nature—this what they call the Dreamtime—whenever you appropriately resonate with the life force.

When I was invited to visit several Aboriginal communities in one of the most remote parts of Australia, I watched the Aborigines pound the earth with their feet in ceremonial dances and move with the rhythmic percussion of clapsticks and the vibratory sound of the didgeridoo. I witnessed how they enter into repetitive natural movements and allow these movements to take over their whole being, sometimes continuing over several days and nights. This brings forth, in their understanding, an opening to the Dreamtime, allowing for an energetic transference to take place between the dancer and the earth.

The Australian Aborigines see the vibratory nature of the universal life force as a realm of flowing energy that engulfs all of life. They call the life force *tumpinyeri mooroop*, which has been translated as "the life spirit of electromagnetic energy."* Aboriginal healing includes the laying on of energized hands. Aboriginal healers know how to tune in to the universal life force and bring its energy into their bodies so that they can then pass it on as a healing current for others. They see themselves tuning in to this energy in a way that is analagous to the way we tune in a radio station.

Aborigines believe that both the human body and the earth itself are magnetically polarized. In the case of the body, the left side typically carries the negative charge while the right side carries the positive charge. Accordingly, when you touch someone with both of your hands, the typical flow of energy is from your right hand to your left hand. Some Aboriginal healers believe that touching the body with your right hand (the positive charge) energizes the spot touched, whereas touching that same spot with your left hand (the negative charge) tends to relax it.

They see the body as interrelated with the magnetic forces of earth, where the energy from the South Pole is the positive source while the North Pole is magnetically negative. When we resonate with the magnetic pulse of the earth, our encapsulated minds become opened and linked with the greater mind of nature. It is this mind that dreams the Dreamtime, the creative force that gives birth to all of reality. Aborigines do see this not as a magical or supernatural occurrence, but as the most natural way you can experience yourself as part of the whole fabric of life.

William Gilbert, the contemporary founder of the science of magnetism, declared that the earth's magnetic field was the soul of the earth. This belief has always been held by the Aborigines. They know

---

*See Cyril Havecker, *Understanding Aboriginal Culture*. Sydney, Australia: Cosmos Periodicals, 1987.

that the vibrations of their being are inseparable from the vibrations of earth and that listening to its voice is the wisest guide to having a vital life.

Aboriginal healers believe that, like a magnet or electrical current that sends its energy waves from positive to negative poles, the thoughts of someone receiving or transmitting the life force must be kept positive, in order to send positive currents of energy into them. Any discordant thoughts that promote fear or worry must be removed, or else the flow of energy will be impeded or distorted. When bringing in the life force, the Aboriginal healer greets its arrival with delight.

I met a remarkable elder Aboriginal healer named Betty Johnston who lives in Halls Creek, an outpost in the Kimberley, the outback land in the northwest corner of Australia. This is one of the most isolated places on the earth, and its exposed sandstone reefs and especially the turrets of a region called the Bungle Bungles remind you that you are in an extremely ancient place. Its hard, brooding landscape formed a natural barrier to invasion, so that the Kimberley nations were undisturbed by European contact until the 1880s. It is one of the few areas in Australia where Aboriginal elders like Betty still live the old ways.

When you are with Betty, she can't keep her hands off of you. She is always hugging, kissing, touching, and even blowing air into you. As she says about herself, "I heal you by loving it right out of you." With an open heart she fills herself with life energy, and then with her body she touches you and moves the life force throughout your whole being, moving out any unnecessary blockages or distress that may have become stuck inside.

This is not simply a physical technique that opens us up to being revitalized by life. We must rid ourselves of ill will, open our hearts, and then wait for the movement that carries us into the energy. In this loving state, we are more naturally tuned to be one with life and to fall into the kind of sympathetic resonance that enables us to be revitalized.

Betty Johnston says she takes a person's illness right into her own heart, but the sick people must have the faith that they can be healed. The kind of faith she is talking about is a feeling of trust that opens you to being more resonant with her. In this trust you drop the fear, worry, negative thoughts, and hopelessness that clog you up and shut you off from receiving the universal life force. Betty uses her body in a powerful way to bring others into a resonance with the force of life. "I have to touch you to know you," Betty is fond of saying. Whether she embraces you with her arms, strokes you with her hands, kisses your body, blows into your mouth, or openly weeps tears upon your head, she fully opens her heart to meet you in the center of the revitalizing and healing resonance.

The Australian medicine man, or *wirinum,* has the ability to enter into a vibrational state that carries him into the highest planes of the spiritual world. There he has access to information that is out of the reach of someone in an ordinary state of mind. As the conductor of ceremony, the *wirinum* sometimes whirls a flat, oval-shaped stick or bullroarer, called a *gayandi,* that creates a whirring, shrieking sound. This sound is a vibration that helps others enter the spiritual realm and find communion with their ancestral spirits. The *wirinum* regards thoughts as well as sounds as creating vibrations that affect our lives. In their sacred ceremonies, Aborigines are fully aware that they are aiming to vibrate with the earth's frequency. Through creating correct thought vibrations they tune themselves to the spiritual force of the universe and are taught, healed, and transformed by it.

Aborigines understand that our thoughts, desires, feelings, and dreams are vibrational forms ready to be energized and subsequently realized. This gives new meaning to what we regard as prayer. Through this perspective, heartfelt prayer is the act of giving life energy to a special thought or request. When we pray with vibrational energy, it may enter into the Dreamtime, where it transcends the common limitations of space and time and sets out to realize itself as part of our reality. This is how prayer can be healing medicine. The Aborigine knows the power that our thoughts can have when they are energized and thrown into the Dreamtime. This is why Aborigines worry when people are careless with their thoughts, feelings, actions, and understanding of nature. If we are out of tune with nature on any level of our being, then we will contribute to throwing the whole ecology into an out-of-tune state, possibly threatening its vitality and its ability to survive.

The Aborigines also respect sexuality as an important way of opening the door to life energy. Both the Aborigines and the African Bushmen believe that we need sex in the same way that we need to breathe and eat. Without it, they propose, we become vulnerable to illness and suffer from a lack of everyday vitality. Sex, when appropriately expressed, is a way to create a relational resonance that vibrates our bodies into the main stream of the life force and fills us with revitalizing energy. The Aborigines live within a network of specifically defined tribal kinship relationships, and sexual encounters outside of their socially defined boundaries are prohibited. Within their social network, however, there is great freedom for sexual expression that sometimes includes public displays, carried out without any sense of sin or shame. There are even highly developed sacred rituals where the community participates in a highly charged communal experience of erotic energy.

The Aborigine's understanding of the vibrational energy fields of life gives them a remarkable relationship with our earth. They can feel the energies of earth and recognize its fatigue when it has supported too much domestic activity. They respect the earth as a living body that requires revitalizing every bit as much as our own bodies. Because of this, the old Aborigine tribes often moved their campsites and rarely stayed in the same place twice. They did not want to tire the land.

Throughout the land they report finding certain energy markings left by the Dreamtime ancestors. These dream trails or tracks are what they call the *songlines* of the Dreamtime. When a group of Aborigines commune with the energy of these places, they believe they are brought into its memory and mind and find themselves able to feel the land and know it in an intimate way. This not only revitalizes their soul; it tunes their whole being to be more in the flow with the natural order of all of life.

Ikuko Osumi, Sensei, and Her Art of Working with Life Energy

Through my travels around the world I encountered different approaches to working with the life force, and I began to wonder how this revitalizing energy could be part of our everyday lives, free and available to all, as it is to the Aborigines of Australia and the Kalahari Bushmen, the oldest cultures on earth. A clue to answering this question came from one of the most extraordinary healers of our time, Ikuko Osumi, Sensei, of Japan. I will tell her story as a way of introducing you to an almost extinct practice of energy work that led me closer to creating the energy technique of Autokinetics.

Years ago, when I first heard about Osumi, Sensei, I felt that I must meet her. Within several weeks I received an invitation to give a keynote address to an anniversary conference on psychotherapy in

Japan.* I wrote to my host and asked for his help in finding Osumi, Sensei. I did not know where she lived, but I suggested that he try to find Dr. Takeshi Hashimoto, who was a professor of anatomy at Toho University Medical School. Dr. Hashimoto had written the foreword to the book by Osumi, Sensei, and Malcolm Ritchie, *The Shamanic Healer: The Healing World of Ikuko Osumi and the Traditional Art of Seiki-Jutsu.*

Unfortunately, my host discovered that Dr. Hashimoto had recently died, and he had no other way to learn where Osumi, Sensei, lived. Then the night before I was to leave for Japan, I received a fax from my host saying that they were delighted to say that they had found her. To their great surprise, she lived right across the street from the university where I would be giving my speech. They had contacted her, and she had agreed to meet me.

I went to Tokyo, gave my speech, and then on the following day was taken to meet Osumi, Sensei. She was a traditional elder woman in her seventies, dressed in a formal kimono. When we first met, she immediately began speaking to me in Japanese, and the translator rushed to keep up with her. She gave an account of my journey around the world, described how I had been initiated into different healing practices, and declared that now it was time for her to teach me how to make all of these different learnings become one truth. She told me that I should cancel my trip home and live with her and she would teach me about *seiki,* the word she used to name the universal life force.

Startled and intrigued by her invitation, I decided to stay a while

---

*Tenth Annual Symposium for the Japanese Association of Family Psychology, Tokyo, Japan, Oct. 30, 1992.

longer in Japan and learn more about this extraordinary woman. I eventually moved into her traditional home, where she and her assistant, Takafumi Okagima, gave me a full transmission of *seiki*. I felt its powerful electrical currents travel through the top of my head to the bottom of my spine. It was the same current of energy I had experienced in ceremonies throughout the world, and it brought forth the natural body movements that I had experienced in my own work with this energy. As I lived with her, she told me the story of her life and taught me what she knew about *seiki*. In her practice, there was an emphasis on becoming an empty vessel so that the energy could flow through you without any distraction. I showed her a film from the Harvard Peabody Museum that documented the Bushmen's healing dance. She was delighted to see how they "transmitted *seiki*," and she saw her own work as essentially the same as what they do under the starlit Kalahari sky. From Osumi, Sensei, I learned to integrate what I had learned from spiritual teachers, shamans, healers, and medicine people from all over the world, and I committed myself to teaching others how the life force may be drawn upon to energize their life.

Seiki is an old Japanese word for life force, and *seiki-jutsu* is the art of working with this force. Ikuko Osumi, Sensei, is one of only a handful of people in the world who are master practitioners of *seiki-jutsu*. Revered as a healer by many of the great artists, cultural teachers, business leaders, and old families of Japan, she devotes herself to giving *seiki* to others.

The work of Ikuko Osumi, Sensei, extends beyond her practice of healing people's symptoms and illnesses. She also has the ability to move the life force into people and teach them how to nurture it on a daily basis. This aspect of her work is of vital importance to anyone who is looking for a practical way to bring more energy and vitality into everyday life. Her life story shows us how her way of working with the life force brings us closer to a simple, practical technique for energizing ourselves.

Born in 1917 in the town of Gamo, Ikuko Osumi grew up in a seashore area about 190 miles north of Tokyo. It was a quiet place where most of the population consisted of fishermen and farmers. As a child she loved to stand on a small mountain called Hiyori and listen to the wind and watch the animals. There she learned about the rhythms of nature and observed how animals and birds treated themselves when they were ill and how plants and animals change in response to different weather conditions.

She was an unusual child who often knew the gender of a baby before it was born and could forecast the weather for the fishing fleets. The local fishermen lived by her word, and she became well-known throughout the surrounding area for her clairvoyance and intuition.

In her midteens, she moved to Tokyo and lived with her aunt and uncle. Because of all of the changes going on in her life, she became quite ill, and she did not respond to any medical treatment. Finally, out of desperation, her aunt tried to do something about her declining health. Osumi, Sensei, described to me what happened during this time in her life:

One afternoon, my aunt called me into the living room and ordered one of the servants to bring tea.

"Ikuko," she said in her somewhat brusque way, "I want you to listen to me. I have something I want to tell you." She stopped and looked directly at me and I lowered my eyes.

She leaned forward. "Every day upstairs at three o'clock, as you probably know well by now," she said, without taking her eyes off me, "I close myself into the three-mat room. The 'exercising' I do is called seiki *exercises. I'm not going to try to explain* seiki *to you now, or go into what kind of exercising it is. All I want to say is that* seiki *is the only thing left that I know can possibly cure you, if you are ever going to get well."*

"If you will do just as I say," she continued after a moment, "I'm sure I can cure you. Are you willing to try?"

What could I say? I nodded my head, without really understanding a thing, or really caring.

She had me sit on a stool in the "seiki room," as she called the room upstairs. She moved behind me, and I couldn't see what she was doing. I do remember that after a while I found myself somehow moving around and around in an endless rocking motion of the body. I somehow related the movement to my fuzzy mental condition at that time. This movement seemed to please my aunt, however, who said that I now had seiki *inside of me.*

It was the next day in the living room that she spoke about what she called the "follow-up" to the instillment of seiki. *"I want you to sit on the stool that's in the seiki room at least once a day for at least ten to twenty minutes. When you sit down put the tips of your fingers together," she said, "and bring them up to your eyes. Touch the balls of your middle and ring fingers against your eyelids. Just wait and see what happens."*

It did sound like nonsense to me, but since my aunt seemed concerned about me, I went dutifully up to the three-mat room and sat down on the seiki stool. I put my fingers together as my aunt had instructed me and proceeded to touch my eyes.

"Hold them there for a time," she had said, so I held them there. Nothing happened, and I felt rather foolish, but then . . . strangely, I found that I was somehow slowly moving in a circular manner, around and around from the hips just as I had done when my aunt

had instilled seiki *in me the day before. Surprised, I let my hands fall to my side and I opened my eyes. The upper part of my body continued to move in a clockwise motion. I had in no way instigated this movement.*

After my first wariness at this unusual, self-propelling movement, I became intrigued and let it move me around and around. It was a most pleasant sensation. My initial apprehension disappeared and I let it move me for the twenty minutes my aunt had spoken of. Then I decided that I had better stop. I did so by stopping the rocking movement through my own will.

"So . . . how did it go?" my aunt inquired when I descended the stairs. I told her exactly what had happened. She seemed very pleased and told me that the next time I did seiki, *I was to touch my body in various places with my hands, rubbing and patting, wherever* seiki *instructed me to place my hands. Those words were indeed strange, but as the days passed, I began to understand what she meant. "Is this what* seiki *is?" I remember wondering to myself, as some force that actually seemed to draw my hand either to my heart or to my eyes, and most often to my lungs. It was strange, yes, but I began to catch a glimpse of just what power my aunt had instilled within me.*

As the days turned into months I found that I began to improve, both physically and mentally. I also began to think that I might become a person like my aunt, who could instill seiki *into others. This was the way I could help other people regain their health . . . I became devoted to the goal of making a career with* seiki.

Ikuko Osumi received *seiki* from her aunt in 1935, and it was the turning point of her life. Once she was filled with *seiki,* the universal life force, she was able to use it in a daily practice that involved natural movements of her body. It was the nurturance of this life energy on a daily basis that brought her health and well-being. As it matured within her, other benefits came forth. She found that her body could be called to touch and energize the bodies of other people. This is how Osumi, Sensei, learned to be a master of *seiki*—by nurturing it within her own body and learning to listen both to its call and to the calls of other bodies.

Osumi, Sensei, believes that the *seiki* in the atmosphere surrounding a person can be amplified and stirred into the form of a vortex. She knows how to concentrate the force in this way and then direct it toward her patients. When she gives a full transmission of *seiki*, she first places the recipient on a wooden bench that is made just for this purpose. She regards the sacrum—the base of the spine—as the site where *seiki* will finally settle, so she relaxes this part of the body before the transmission begins.

As she readies herself to transmit the energy, she feels a heavy, abundant flow of *seiki* gathering from every direction. She attracts and gathers this energy by making spontaneous loud vocal noises and by banging on the walls. She then falls into a special state of consciousness in which she feels no distinction between her body and mind and subsequently "becomes absorbed into the body of her client," as she puts it.

When the time feels right, she places her hands above the head of the recipient and allows the accumulated energy to flow naturally into his or her body. The *seiki* moves into the recipient through the top of the head, where it sometimes feels like a slight electrical shock. It slowly travels down the neck and spine, finally resting in the sacrum. The patient usually starts to rock back and forth at this time, and this rocking is taken as a sign that the person has received *seiki*. In this process, the giver and receiver feel as though they have become one body, and they jointly bring forth a natural rhythmic motion. The time to receive *seiki* varies from person to person, as does the form of rhythm and motion that is bestowed.

I was able to be present with Osumi, Sensei, when she worked with her clients, and she allowed me to interview them and hear their stories about how *seiki* had affected their lives. I watched her teach how they could bring the life force into their own bodies and how this daily practice brought health and vitality to their lives. Her clients included the director of the National Noh Theater and the renowned scientist Dr. Toshi Doi, who invented the compact disk and who now has a laboratory designed for the study of the life force.

Osumi, Sensei, took me to the corporate headquarters of Sony to meet Dr. Toshi Doi. He told us how the scientific measurement of *ki* or *seiki* would be the greatest scientific contribution of the next century. Although several Nobel Prize–winning scientists had worked on this problem, he felt that we were at least ten years away from measuring and scientifically validating the life force and expressing it in the mathematics required for the scientific community to accept it. He already believed that Einstein's work was missing the presence of the *ki* factor and that the introduction of this notion into his equations would result in paradigm-shifting scientific breakthroughs.

Several years after my first visit to Japan, Osumi, Sensei, came to my home in the United States and watched me do energy work with dozens of people, including her own daughter, Masako, a contemporary artist in Tokyo who accompanied her on the trip. She then had me assist her in giving *seiki* to my eleven-year-old son. We accumulated the life force over his head, and I could actually feel it become a taffy-like substance, something that could be touched and spread over his head. When he received it, his body began to rock and move naturally.

More than a year later Osumi, Sensei, sent me a fax saying that she must immediately come back to the United States. She had something to say that had to be said in person. The following week she and her daughter and a family friend arrived, and when we gathered for a meal, she told the story of how she had first dedicated her life to the practice of *seiki-jutsu*. At that time she went to the shrine of an ancestor and was given a piece of wood on which she inscribed her name and personal pledge. She knew that someday she would give this piece of wood to one of her successors. She then paused in telling her story, reached down to take a piece of wood from her bag, and handed it to me, saying, "I have placed your name on this wood next to my name. You are now to tell everyone about how people may bring *seiki*, the universal life force, into their everyday life."

The Future of Energy Healing

Every mystical practice in the world seems to have discovered the spiritually empowering contribution of a direct encounter with the life force. These spiritual traditions include not only the ones discussed here, but also Celtics, Greeks, Tibetans, Hawaiians, cabbalists, early gnostics, Freemasons, theosophists, and Latin Americans, to name a few. In contemporary times, work with this energy has taken place among some Western schools of psychotherapy and specialized forms of body work and consciousness training. Some of these stem from the work of the psychotherapist Wilhelm Reich, who discussed the life force in terms of "orgone energy" and found that health and well-being were brought about by activating and expressing this energy in the body.

Other Western approaches that help awaken the flow of the life force, such as Rolfing and polarity therapy, were influenced by the hands-on practice of osteopathy, founded by a mid-nineteenth-century physician, Dr. Andrew Still. The original form of osteopathy was a true Hippocratic medicine based on touching and moving the body. The adjustment of bones, the well-known bone cracking accomplished by classic osteopaths and chiropractors, results in an immediate flow of energy in the body. This takes place as the space between the bones is shifted, allowing for a moment when the body feels as if it has entered a kind of gravity-free space. This brief experience gives the patient an encounter with the flow of the life force.

At their center, all therapies of body movement, from osteopathy to Rolfing, Alexander, and Feldenkrais, involve this introduction to the universal force of life. Without knowing it, these Western approaches found the same general truth as other healing traditions around the world. History will show, I am convinced, that the early discoveries of osteopathy and other related practices were among the most important contributions of Western culture to the healing arts. The leading contemporary philosopher of the body, Don Hanlon Johnson, underscores how the invention of different body therapies arises from the originator's own spontaneous movements, which too easily become rigidified when they become formalized and taught to others in an authoritative manner. The most promising future for body work will be more in the direction of returning us to an experience of basic, natural movements that take place effortlessly and spontaneously. These movements, which are linked with our internal rhythms—cellular, circulatory, respiratory, lymphatic, peristalic, nervous, and micromuscular—move us to be moved at the most primal level of awareness and being. This is the heart and soul of all indigenous healing practices, and it is what Autokinetics is all about.

I also want to mention the pioneering work of Dr. David Akstein, one of the acknowledged founders of medical hypnosis in Brazil. He studied the healing rites of indigenous cultures, particularly the frenzied dance rituals of the South American Umbanda religion. His research led to the discovery of a unique form of trance, which he called the "kinetic trance," brought about by the moving body of someone involved in ceremonial dancing. This trance is similar to the "tuning zone" of Autokinetics.

Dr. Akstein and I have shared our work with one another, and he enthusiastically supports what I am presenting to you. Since both of us have learned from indigenous healers and have elaborated ways of using automatic body movement to induce special states of consciousness that have therapeutic benefits, Dr. Akstein calls me his "spiritual son."

In *Spontaneous Healing,* Dr. Andrew Weil devotes a chapter to the remarkable healing gifts of Dr. Robert Fulford, a warm and caring osteopath who knew how to move the life force through the bodies of those who came to him for treatment. Dr. Weil wrote the foreword to Dr. Fulford's book on the natural life force and proclaimed that "if medicine is to come back into alignment with the great healing traditions and satisfy the needs and desires of those who are sick, it must recover the truths that Bob Fulford expresses."

Dr. Fulford and I were friends and colleagues. When he was ninety-one years old, we had several opportunities to touch one another and exchange the life force. He was enthusiastic about Autokinetics and was delighted with its simplicity and ability to bring the life force into daily life.

Dr. Fulford passed away on June 26, 1997. I end this book with a special dedication to the gentle wisdom and healing power that this caring doctor gave to the world. He was a genuine inspiration, and he wanted everyone to know how the life force can vitalize the body, spirit, and intellect. With his special encouragement and endorsement, I was more deeply moved to write this book.

As scientists continue to validate the positive results of energy healing, we ourselves must become aware of the benefits that come from moving with the life force. Dr. Robert Becker, author of *The Body Electric* and professor of orthopedics at the Upstate Medical Center in Syracuse, New York, declares, "Later in history, this will be judged to have been the primary discovery of the twentieth century, . . . that is, that the human organism is sensitive to electro-magnetic fields, that it produces its own electro-magnetic fields, that electrical currents flow through the organism, and that in all of this we are part of the living process of the entire cosmos."

Of course, this discovery has been made by all indigenous people throughout the world since the beginning of human history. We are simply the last people to get the word about life energy. Perhaps our greatest hope for the future depends not only on recognizing the force that is life, but on learning how to bring it into our bodies. In so doing, we will become closer to life itself. This newfound intimacy with nature, I believe, will bring us closer to one another. Then we can dance to the rhythm of earth's heart underneath the light of a moon that whispers its secrets to our primitively awakened souls.

SUGGESTED READING

Akstein, David, *Un Voyage à Travers la Transe*. Paris: Éditions Sand, 1992.

Barnett, H. G., *Indian Shakers*. Carbondale: Southern Illinois University Press, 1957.

Bateson, Gregory, and Margaret Mead, *Balinese Character: A Photographic Analysis*. New York: New York Academy of Sciences, 1942.

Becker, Robert O., *The Body Electric: Electromagnetism and the Foundation of Life*. New York: Morrow, 1985.

Benor, Daniel, *Healing Research: Holistic Energy Medicine and Spiritual Healing*, Volume 1, London: Helix Editions, 1993.

Benson, Herbert, *The Relaxation Response*. New York: Morrow, 1975.

Brennan, Barbara Ann, *Hands of Light: A Guide to Healing Through the Human Energy Field*. New York: Bantam, 1988.

Bruyere, Rosalyn L., *Wheels of Light: A Study of the Chakras*. (Jeanne Farrens, ed.) Sierra Madre, Calif.: Bon Productions, 1989.

Burr, Harold Saxton, *Blueprint for Immortality: The Electric Patterns of Life*. Essex, England: Daniel, 1972.

Cleary, Thomas, *Vitality, Energy, Spirit*. Boston: Shambhala, 1991.

Cohen, Kenneth S., *The Way of Qigong: The Art and Science of Chinese Energy Healing*. New York: Ballantine Books, 1997.

Dossey, Larry, *Healing Words: The Power of Prayer and the Practice of Medicine*. San Francisco: Harper, 1993.

————. *Prayer Is Good Medicine*. San Francisco: Harper, 1996.

————. *Recovering the Soul: A Scientific and Spiritual Search*. New York: Bantam, 1989.

Eisenberg, David, with Thomas Lee Wright, *Encounters with Qi: Exploring Chinese Medicine*. New York: Bantam, 1989.

Erickson, Milton H., *The Collected Papers of Milton H. Erickson on Hypnosis*, Ernest L. Rossi, ed. New York: Irvington, 1980.

Evans, F. W., *Shakers: Compendium of the Origin, History, Principles, Rules and Regulations, Government, and Doctrines of the United Society of Believers in Christ*. New York, 1859.

Ford, Clyde W., *Where Healing Waters Meet: Touching Mind and Emotion Through the Body*. Barrytown, N.Y.: Station Hill, 1989.

Fulford, Robert C., *Dr. Fulford's Touch of Life: The Healing Power of the Natural Life Force.* New York: Pocket Books, 1996.

Gerber, Richard, *Vibrational Medicine.* Santa Fe, N. Mex.: Bear, 1988.

Grossinger, Richard, *Planet Medicine: Modalities.* Berkeley, Calif.: North Atlantic, 1995.

Hallowell, A. Irving, *The Role of Conjuring in Salteaux Society.* Philadelphia: University of Pennsylvania Press, 1942.

Harpur, Tom, *The Uncommon Touch: An Investigation of Spiritual Healing.* Toronto, Canada: McClelland and Stewart, 1994.

Havecker, Cyril, *Understanding Aboriginal Culture.* Sydney, Australia: Cosmos Periodicals, 1987.

Herrigel, Eugen, *Zen in the Art of Archery.* New York: Pantheon, 1953.

Hunt, Valerie V., *Infinite Mind: The Science of Human Vibrations.* Malibu, Calif.: Malibu Publishing, 1995.

Johnson, Don Hanlon, ed., *Body, Spirit, and Democracy.* Berkeley, Calif.: North Atlantic Books, 1993.

————. *Bone, Breath, and Gesture: Practices of Embodiment.* Berkeley, Calif.: North Atlantic Books, 1995.

Katz, Richard, *Boiling Energy: Community Healing Among the Kalahari Kung.* Cambridge, Mass.: Harvard University Press, 1982.

Keeney, Bradford, *Everyday Soul: Awakening the Spirit in Daily Life.* New York: Riverhead, 1996.

Krieger, Dolores, *Therapeutic Touch: How to Use Your Hands to Help or to Heal.* Englewood Cliffs, N.J.: Prentice-Hall, 1979.

————. "The Relationship of Touch, with Intent to Help or Heal, to Subjects' In-vivo Hemoglobin Values: A Study in Personalized Interaction," Proceedings, American Nurses Association Ninth Nursing Research Conference, San Antonio, Texas, March 21–23, 1973, pp. 39–58.

Krippner, Stanley, and Patrick Welch, *Spiritual Dimensions of Healing: From Native Shamanism to Contemporary Health Care.* New York: Irvington, 1992.

Larsen, Stephen, *The Shaman's Doorway: Opening Imagination to Power and Myth.* Barrytown, N.Y.: Station Hill, 1988.

Lawlor, Robert, *Voices of the First Day: Awakening in the Aboriginal Dreamtime.* Rochestor, Vt.: Inner Traditions, 1991.

McGaa, Ed, *Mother Earth Spirituality: Native American Paths to Healing Ourselves and Our World.* San Francisco: Harper, 1990.

Miner, Malcolm, *Your Touch Can Heal: A Guide to Healing Touch and How to Use It.* Keswick, Va.: Faith Ridge, 1990.

Mookerjee, Ajit, *Kundalini: The Arousal of the Inner Energy.* Rochester, Vt.: Destiny Books, 1991.

Mooney, James, *The Ghost-Dance Religion and Wounded Knee.* n.p,: Dover, 1973.

Mutwa, Vusamazulu Credo, *Song of The Stars: The Lore of a Zulu Songoma.* Stephen Larsen, ed. Barrytown, N.Y.: Station Hill, 1996.

Myss, Caroline, *Anatomy of the Spirit: The Seven Stages of Power and Healing.* New York: Harmony, 1996.

Ni, Maoshing, *The Yellow Emperor's Classic of Medicine,* Boston, Mass.: Shambhala, 1995.

Osumi, Ikuko, and Malcolm Ritchie, *The Shamanic Healer: The Healing World of Ikuko Osumi and the Traditional Art of Seiki-Jutsu.* Rochester, Vt.: Healing Arts Press, 1988.

Pagels, Elaine, *The Gnostic Gospels.* New York: Vintage, 1979.

Pollack, Andrew, "The Life Force in the Briefcase," *The New York Times,* November 28, 1995 (feature essay in "Business Day"), pp. C1–C3.

Powers, William, *Yuwipi: Vision and Experience in Oglala Ritual.* Lincoln: University of Nebraska Press, 1982.

Sannella, Lee, *The Kundalini Experience.* Lower Lake, Calif.: Integral, 1987.

Schwarz, Jack, *The Human Energy System.* New York: Dutton, 1980.

Shih, Tzu Kuo, *Qi Gong Therapy: The Chinese Art of Healing with Energy.* Barrytown, N.Y.: Station Hill, 1994.

Thomas, Lewis, *The Lives of a Cell.* New York: Viking, 1974.

Tucker, Michael, *Dreaming With Open Eyes: The Shamanic Spirit in Twentieth Century Art and Culture.* London: Aquarian/Thorsons, 1992.

van der Post, Laurens, *The Creative Pattern in Primitive Africa.* Dallas, Tex.: Spring, 1957.

Weil, Andrew, *Spontaneous Healing.* New York: Knopf, 1995.

ABOUT THE AUTHOR

Bradford Keeney, Ph.D., is a much sought-after keynote speaker who conducts workshops throughout the world. He is vice president of cultural affairs for the Ringing Rocks Foundation, and his most recent popular book was *Everyday Soul: Awakening the Spirit in Daily Life*. Dr. Keeney is also an internationally renowned teacher of psychotherapy who has written several academic books that are deemed classics in the field of family therapy. He has directed several clinical doctoral programs and has worked at some of the most respected psychotherapy centers in the United States, including the Ackerman Institute in New York City, the Karl Menninger Center in Topeka, and the Philadelphia Child Guidance Clinic at the University of Pennsylvania.